Nutriti... ...nd
Athletic
Performance

"Using Dr. Graham's program and his special sports drinks, there is no end to my endurance."
—Rudy Carti, World Record Holder,
151,000 abdominal crunches in 48 hours

"Every aspect of my performance has improved. After two years on Dr. Graham's program, I found myself in the best shape of my life—my speed drills faster than ever and also my recovery."
—Ronnie Grandison,
Veteran NBA Basketball Player

"Before Dr. Graham's program, I swam for twenty-two hours and couldn't get across. After Dr. Graham's program, I made the crossing in eleven hours and had enough energy left over to return by kayak. It took only seven more hours."
—Kenny Croes,
The first and only person to swim the "impossible"
Aruba to the Venezuela crossing

"My energy has soared. I recover faster, and my sore muscles went away."
—Nancy Martin,
Professional Snowboarder

"I ski harder, recover faster, am quicker, and have more power."
—Len Smith,
Ski Instructor

"Now my skateboard wears out before I do!"
—Ador Lazar,
Professional Skateboarder

Nutrition and Athletic Performance:

A Handbook for Athletes and Fitness Enthusiasts

by

Dr. Douglas N. Graham

Nutrition and Athletic Performance

http://www.foodnsport.com

Revised from Nutrition and Athletic Performance,
Copyright 1999, 2008.
All rights reserved.

Cover photos by Elan Sunstar.

ISBN 978-1-893831-08-7 • $17.95

Athletes have been eating whole fruit since the beginning of recorded history. The body requires a wide assortment of nutrients to healthfully metabolize calories. Fruit is great fuel!

DEDICATION

This book is dedicated to every athlete with whom I have worked and to each person, athlete or not, who gives this time-proven program a chance to work. May your health and your physical performance soar to new heights and surpass your imagined limits.

TABLE OF CONTENTS

ACKNOWLEDGMENTS

I count myself fortunate to have had so many excellent teachers. To all of you who have played a part in my life's education, I extend my sincerest and most heartfelt thanks. From the beginning, my parents, Marty and Bea, have been my best teachers and greatest supporters. I also want to thank my sister, Nissan Graham-Mayk. She has looked out for me for a lifetime, helped me on countless projects, and contributed in a big way to the editing of this book. I give a huge thanks as well to my angel, my wife, Rozi, who ceaselessly read and reread this manual for content, meaning, clarity, and technical correctness.

As I contemplate my physical education along the way, I think first of Olympic swimmer John Cittadino and all his staff at Seashore Day Camp who instilled a love of sports in me that has never waned. Gus Villapiano Sr. helped me overcome my intense fear of water and eventually become a water safety instructor trainer. Jim Asbell, my first health and physical education teacher, gave me a great appreciation for the gifts of health, fitness, teamwork, and competition. Olympic champion gymnast Dr. Joseph Toth, who was my college gymnastics coach, explained the role of physics in gymnastics and gave me a better understanding of hard work. National champion gymnast Dr. Terry Orlick helped me understand how to meld performing art with sport via the trampoline. World champion trampolinist Dan Millman taught me the joy and value of trampoline's "diddly moves." George Hery, another champion trampolinist, unknowingly filled in the missing pieces for me in a lecture/performance he gave one afternoon that provided me the insight to teach movement skills in tiny parts. This insight eventually enabled each of the seven children on my tiny trampoline team to win a national championship in 1980. And so my education continued. A special thanks to Dr. V. V. Vetrano and Ron Weston, both lifetime devotees of hygienic living, who, through their own example, reinforced my belief that a raw food diet is the ultimate program for all athletes.

I sincerely want to thank all of the teachers who invested their time and energy into my education. I remember all of you, by name, and each of you played an important role in allowing me to develop into the person that I am today.

For the second edition of this book, I would lastly like to thank Lennie Mowris. The research you provided and the time you took to help this book reach its full potential will not be forgotten.

FOREWORD

Nutrition and Athletic Performance: A Handbook for Athletes and Fitness Enthusiasts holds within its pages a quality of information that is both rare and of immeasurable value. Athletes do not need yet another complex "authoritative" text on a subject that is already in a state of analytical paralysis. What is needed is an entirely new approach to nutrition that puts the fragmented thinking back together. Dr. Graham teaches effective sports nutrition with elegant simplicity. He takes the hand of the reader and guides step-by-step toward the superior daily food choices that make the difference between athletic participation and athletic excellence.

True athleticism is the celebration of physical life. It is the platform upon which the miracle of nature expresses her human exuberance. Lucky are those who have found the inspiration needed to fuel the fire of their own recreational play, for they will reap the rewards of greater health and joy. Those few who have been gifted with the talent and opportunity to secure an income by participating in the physical theater we call "professional sports" may consider themselves blessed.

Since the infancy of the written word, "health" and "athleticism" have been referred to in a symbiotic and interchangeable way. In recent times, however, the collective academic brain has given birth to a technological age whose influence has spun out of control and infiltrated aspects of human existence, causing perversion and destruction. This scientific mayhem is ripping apart healthy athletes and replacing them with a kaleidoscope of genetically engineered parts.

The void that exists between an individual's desire to reach a goal and the willingness to make the personal changes necessary to achieve those goals is becoming wider and deeper. The expansion of this "dead space" is predominately the result of an ever-increasing belief that science and technology may be held responsible for personal success, replacing the intrinsic self-discipline and committed application demonstrated by our ancestors.

Technology is not evil. On the contrary, it is the inevitable outcome of our human search for information about ourselves and the complex planet upon which we live. Similar to money, which is innocuous enough in itself, the degree to which technology is useful or destructive lies in direct accordance with its application.

However, today's approach to sports nutrition is an example of technological misuse. In our attempt to dissect and analyze the laws of nature and physics, we have sacrificed other levels of our awareness. We have lost sight of the fact that the entire complexity of all life-forms, from the single-celled organelle to entire ecosystems, is far greater than the sum of its component parts. We have paid the price for our curiosity in ways that have yet to be appreciated.

This fragmented approach to science has permeated virtually all aspects of education, but none more so than that related to athletic performance. Hot on the heels of scientific endeavor rides the jockey of marketing, whose game it is to supply products and then create a demand for them. Comparable to patients who consume medicines prescribed by their medical doctors without knowing the causes of their ailments or the implications of their drugs, many athletes spend vast amounts of money on nutritional supplements that they neither understand nor need. The remaining sports people either choose to be oblivious to the implications of nutrition upon their performance or are rendered unable to improve their diets by the total confusion of conflicting information they are fed.

Theoretical understanding of any subject, however, is only the precursor to practical application. Your athletic performance and health experience will not be affected one iota just by reading this book. Your potential can only be realized by weaving Dr. Graham's recommendations into the fabric of your training. Any concept remains a belief or disbelief, and does not qualify for judgment until it is directly experienced in the fullness of its reality. I encourage you to read, apply, and only then, evaluate, this information. I am confident that anyone who does this in earnest will come to consider this little handbook the most valuable book on sports nutrition they will ever read.

Professor Rozalind A. Gruben, AHSI, RSA

INTRODUCTION

This book is for everyone: world-class athletes who hope to reach their fullest potential, the coaches and trainers who work with them, and the everyday fitness enthusiasts who wish to excel. It is meant for those who feel the frustration of doling out their top performances in short bursts, a few minutes here and a few moments there, who would rather be on top of their game at all times. It is designed to allow athletes to focus on being athletes; giving them the freedom to eat well without having to worry about chemistry, nutrition, or the inconvenience of indigestion. It is intended to help sports-minded people see beyond the marketing of products, the hype of advertising, the trendy but inevitably disappointing diets, gimmicks, flushes, cleanses, super-foods, and supplements. Every athlete, without exception, who has applied the principles outlined in this book, has achieved superb results. With a little practice and persistence, *you* can too.

Most books on nutrition turn out to be rather complicated and confusing chemistry books. They refer to isolated nutrients rather than whole foods. They cite research, provide graphs, utilize many charts and tables, but never quite give the information one is looking for. In this book, I have made an effort to minimize number crunching, the religion of nutrition, and rely, instead, on common-sense applications of basic nutritional facts. True nutrition should be more than a bunch of formulas tied to mumbo-jumbo about micrograms, millimoles, kilocalories, joules, and partially-hydrogenated polyunsaturated esters. It should be the logical application of what we know to be true about ourselves combined with the basics facts about our food. Nutrition teachers that rely upon wowing you with long words and phrases that you have never heard of, and confusing you with concepts that you aren't even sure make any sense at all, will never free you to make your own, sound, nutritional decisions. They aren't truly functioning as teachers at all, whose purpose is to free you to be able to think for yourself, but are, instead, attempting to become gurus with a large following of devotees, dealers of products that they can sell to their customer base, and jailers of the mind, body, and spirit.

The fragmented vision used by many nutritionists allows them to recommend things that don't make sense. A daily small quantity of alcohol, a protoplasmic poison that kills any and all living cells with which it comes into contact, is recommended because it has been found that its consumption on a regular basis lowers blood pressure. But what about the damage it does to the brain, liver, health, and vitality? How can the damage caused by alcohol consumption be ignored simply because it can be used to treat one symptom of unhealthful living? Throughout the animal kingdom, healthful living and eating practices result in normal healthy blood pressure. Why shouldn't this principle work for us as well?

In this book, I teach you how to create health through participation in healthy habits, to minimize symptoms by removing their cause(s), rather than how to treat, suppress, deal with, and live with symptoms by using food (or worse, the isolated nutrients in food) medicinally.

A philosophical approach to healthful eating encourages us to eat only those foods to which we are biologically adapted, one type at a time, and only when hungry. This method is practiced in the wild by every animal on the planet. Healthful eating teaches us to eat until satiated—never overeating and never becoming fat. The value of a food should not be judged by the amount of advertising it receives, how exciting or novel it is, or what its traditional use has been, but by its ability to satiate without stimulating, subduing, drugging, irritating, or outright harming its eaters. In the words of my old friend and mentor, health reformer T. C. Fry, "The Golden Rule of Eating is: Thou shalt not poison thyself." No one should have to recover from a meal!

Chapter One
NUTRITIONAL CLARITY

It is my intention to clear the smoke from the field of nutrition, metaphorically speaking, and make sound nutritional choices simple for anyone, athlete or not, who wants to eat the best foods available. This makes nutrition understandable and easy, allowing people to sanely and healthfully take their nutrition into their own hands. Those making a living in any field related to human nutrition may view this as blasphemy against the status quo. To them, I can only quote the words of the late Herbert M. Shelton, D.C., "Let us have the truth, though the heavens may fall."

Athletes around the world are notorious for trying every nutritional regimen imaginable to boost their physical performance. Billions of dollars and man-hours are spent in research to define the role of human nutrition in relationship to physical performance. Nutrition and sports performance laboratories in almost every university add to the search for even the smallest nutritional advantage to be gained by today's athlete. All this exhaustive study focuses mainly on discovering nutrients that can be added to the diet for positive effect. Little or no study has been done to locate nutrient factors that would have a positive effect on physical performance if they were subtracted from the diet. Almost no research has been done to find out what happens to sports performance when people eat according to their anatomical and physiological nature, but interestingly, the research that has been done has all been extremely promising and positive.

It is interesting to note that although sports records have improved dramatically over the past five decades due mainly to sophistications in training techniques and technological advances, human nutrition has deteriorated, for the most part, in all sectors of the population. Since the end of World War II, thousands of toxic chemical pesticides, herbicides, fungicides, insecticides, rodenticides, steroidal drugs, preservatives, coloring agents, flavor enhancers, and growth hormones have been introduced into, and onto, our food supply. The result of modern food chemistry has been detrimental for all human health, not to mention its negative effects on athletic performance.

Scientists have stretched and twisted technology, sometimes to the point of the bizarre, in their attempts to evaluate the role of various nutrients in enhancing athletic performance. Almost every known nutritive substance has been studied in exhaustive detail. Nutrients, weather conditions, training strategies, various medical tricks such as blood doping, differing competition scenarios—all these have been subjected to comprehensive examination in the effort to help athletes upgrade their performance. Yet for the most part, these efforts have produced no truly helpful results. And rarely in these studies has the overall health, career longevity, or quality of life for the athlete been a primary consideration. In our quest to reach the ultimate in physical performance, we must always remember that athletes are, first and foremost, individual people with personal lives to lead outside of their sports career. To help them perform better at sports while compromising their health should never be a viable option.

> Athletes will try almost anything to boost their performance. Why won't they give healthful living serious consideration? Perhaps because it implies too much personal responsibility?

It is relatively simple for science to demonstrate that a lack of certain nutrients will lead to serious health problems, sometimes even death. It follows, therefore, that a lack of certain nutrients can result in lowered physical performance. One of the first symptoms of a sports-related nutrient insufficiency is a feeling of deep tiredness. Low levels of sodium, potassium, iron, water and/or blood sugar can leave an athlete feeling rundown.

Symptoms of vitamin insufficiencies are relatively rare in today's athletes. Fresh fruits and vegetables, the best sources of these nutrients, make up a larger portion of an athlete's diet today than they did years ago when vitamin-deficiency diseases such as rickets, scurvy, and beriberi were common.

> The concept of "better living through chemistry" has been debunked time and again. The International Olympic Committee frowns on the use of performance-enhancing drugs. Still, athletes mistakenly look to the needle to inject their success, rather than ingesting it on their forks.

Inadequate levels of protein consumption are also uncommon and an insufficiency of fat is all but unknown. A diet lacking in carbohydrate is still a major nutritional issue, however, as is the type of carbohydrate that should be consumed for optimal performance.

Interestingly, little research has been done to demonstrate the performance problems associated with the oversufficiency of various nutrients. Too many calories will result in an overfat athlete, no matter how those calories are consumed, whether in the form of protein, fat, or carbohydrate. It is also possible to cause severe harm—even death—through the overconsumption of the fat soluble vitamins A, D, E, and K. Minerals can be a problem, too, if they are taken in excess or in an inorganic form which the body can-

> When we look to individual nutrients to boost athletic performance, we look in error. Instead, we must look to whole foods.

not use. This can result in electrolyte and other imbalances, as well as kidney problems.

Nutritional research is funded primarily by the manufacturers of supplements and prepared foods. Because of this, as the sciences of chemistry and nutrition "advance," our foods are fragmented and refined into increasingly smaller segments, and are then marketed according to the nutrients in them, rather than the quality of the foods themselves. This processing of foods into their component parts tends to be satisfying for chemists and financially rewarding for the companies that sell the resulting supplements, but it is done to the health and nutrition detriment of the consumer.

With the health of the consumer in decline, scientists easily find new grant money to justify the "progress" of experimenting with every fraction of foodstuff that is discovered. It is interesting to note that when barely a hundred nutrients were known to man, it was estimated that there might be as many as three hundred in existence. Now that several hundred thousand nutrients are known, it is estimated there are at least a hundred thousand left to find.

Sadly, most experimentation in nutrition is geared toward proving the value of this or that nutrient factor extracted from a specific food or food group and often taken in mega doses. This "scientific" approach is actually backward when compared to the way people were born to eat. The human body was designed to consume whole foods, not individual nutrients.

> What athletes need is higher quality food, not higher quality supplements.

Unexpected results keep popping up when experiments are performed to show the positive effects of isolated nutrient factors on the human body. Substance "A" is found in one group of vegetables, for example, and it is shown to have certain special qualities. Let's say, for the sake of argument, that substance "A" helps prevent cancer. Therefore, when substance "A" is isolated and consumed by a control group in a scientific study, a reduction in certain types of cancers would be expected. Unfortunately, it's not that simple and frequently no reduction in cancer is found at all. This phenomenon can be attributed to as yet undiscovered factors in the world of nutrition. Some unknown component must work in combination with substance "A" for it to be effective in fighting cancer. All this leaves us in the uncomfortable position of trusting scientists to produce reliable results when there are at least nine strikes against them:

1. The scientist usually is hired to prove the value of a certain nutrient(s), rather than to discover the truth about that nutrient.

2. The scientist is hired by a company with vested financial interests in the "positive" results of that scientist's experiments. S/he is obligated to word and state the results accordingly, in order to please the employer. Many of these companies already have a profound history of misrepresenting the "facts" and misleading the public.

3. People naturally want to eat foods for pleasure and nutrition rather than consuming pills for the same benefit. Because of this inborn trait, the results of "scientific" tests are often presented in a misleading light with the intention of fostering emotional dependence on the consumption of supplements.

4. Extracting nutrients from whole foods, processing them, and then selling them as food supplements is the most costly way to bring nutrients to the marketplace. It can cost the consumer a great deal more to purchase a variety of supplements than it would cost to obtain the same nutrients directly from whole foods.

5. Supplementation is an inadequate and incomplete method of supplying nutrients because it is impossible to match nature's delicate mix and balance of nutrition.

6. There has never been a successful attempt at keeping an animal or person healthy, or even simply alive, on a diet composed strictly of nutritional supplements.

7. With an estimated 60 to 90 percent (the number depends upon whom

> Selling supplements is a brilliant marketing idea, but it is not nutritionally sound. Only whole foods supply all the nutrients you need to perform at your physical peak.

you use as your source) of all vital nutrients in food as yet undiscovered, why should we add nutrients one at a time to our diets, or expect that any nutritional supplementation program could possibly be "complete"? Why not simply eat whole foods?

8. Most nutrients are known to interact symbiotically with at least eight other nutrients. This makes the odds of supplying any one individual nutrient in a healthful manner infinitesimally small. It is simply impossible to get the dosage and ratio correct, except through the consumption of whole foods.

9. Based on past experience, we must consider the reliability of the "nutrients discovered" estimate to be incredibly low. As we are discovering more nutrients all the time, it is more likely that something as low as 1 percent of all nutrients has been found to date and named by our scientific community. Again, in this light, comprehensive nutritional supplementation must be viewed as anything but comprehensive.

On the positive side, certain basic facts have not changed since the first investigations into the controversial field of nutrition:

- Fruits still provide the highest percentage of vitamins per calorie consumed, with vegetables coming in second.
- Vegetables still provide the highest percentage of minerals per calorie consumed, with fruits coming in second.
- The nutritional makeup of fruit is closest to mimicking human nutritional needs of any food, and vegetables are second.
- Almost every vegetable that can be eaten whole, fresh, and raw contains all eight of the essential amino acids (as do most fruits) and, therefore, provides us with complete protein. (There are 20 amino acids involved in human

nutrition. According to current scientific thought, eight of these can only be supplied through our foods while the other 12 can be synthesized by the liver.)

- A random mix of fruits will provide about the same percentage of protein per calorie as found in mother's milk. This is certainly an adequate amount of protein, even for an adult human.
- A random mix of vegetables will provide about four to five times the RDA of protein per calorie consumed.
- Plant foods contain essentially no cholesterol and, overall, are renowned for their health value.

The obvious conclusion to be drawn from the above scenario is that there is only one path to the very best nutrition: eat fresh, ripe, whole, raw, organic plant foods. Humankind has relied on such foods for nutritional vitality since the beginning of its tenure on planet Earth.

According to most anthropologists, human beings have relied on a diet comprised almost exclusively of whole, fresh, ripe, raw, organic fruits and vegetables for at least the first 99.9 percent of our history. This sane determination is deficient in only one aspect. It does not support the creation of an ever-more complex, isolated, and indecipherable field of study called nutritional science. It also does not create an overdependence on nutritionists, dietitians, food scientists, food chemists, and specialized doctors to make healthful eating a reality. Instead, it takes the entire field of nutrition and makes it little more than common sense. It encourages athletes and nonathletes alike to think for themselves and frees them to consume the foods they were born to eat.

> Increase the percentage of whole, fresh, ripe, raw, organic, fruits and vegetables in your diet and know that you are heading in the healthiest possible direction.

Chapter Two
OPTIMUM ATHLETIC RECOVERY

As an integral part of vibrant health, high levels of physical fitness offer many rewarding opportunities. People who enjoy the physical side of life find that vigorous activity can be wonderfully pleasing. The personal growth, improvement in performance, and mental strength that develop with dedicated practice and animated play often provide a great sense of satisfaction. A feeling of connectedness with others develops both through team play and in the knowledge that many people around the world participate in these same activities. The lessons learned in physical

> For optimum performance, foods with negative effects must be eliminated from the diet.

training can be applied to all walks of life. These lessons include patience, persistence, goal setting, repetition, and teamwork. It is quite common to find that a high percentage of the most successful businesspeople had a long and committed investment in sports before they began their business careers.

Part of the maturation process is that we become aware of our physical limitations. Another part, which many people consider to be the fun part of life, is that we also gain the knowledge and expertise to push ourselves to the edge of those limits. Being active as regularly as we want can prove to be a challenge, however, and recovery from this activity can be slower than expected. The "weekend warrior" is not the only one at risk in this scenario. Because most of us fall into routines that rarely vary, we consistently overtrain some muscle groups while undertraining others. Though we may be fit for our sport, having trained specific muscle groups, we are likely not fit for activities that call more heavily upon muscle groups that we do not typically train. The runner who goes for a biking weekend, the soccer player who swims and surfs for the first time in years, and the once-a-year skier are all at risk. Sore joints, stiff muscles, lethargy, and acute injuries are a few of the initial symptoms of the overtraining syndrome.

Sports scientists, fitness trainers, athletes, and coaches put tremendous quantities of time and energy into improving training techniques. Cross training, weight training, build-up and taper-down strategies, phased training, and specificity of workouts have all contributed to the perpetual breaking of athletic records and to the increased intensity of team and individual sports. The "impossible" 4-minute mile is now a common event, run not only by world-class milers but by high school boys and even a few men over 40 years of age. Women's sports records are falling even faster than men's.

> The number of records being broken is amazing.
> The number of athletes being broken is even more amazing.

Training harder does not always translate into training smarter, however, nor does it guarantee results. Sports injuries, both mild and severe, acute and chronic, are at an all-time high. It is not uncommon for burnout to hit young athletes before they ever reach their prime.

The number of athletic careers that end due to injury before they ever really got started is absolutely amazing. Many professional sports are now dominated by teenagers. The 30-year-old athlete is becoming a rarity in gymnastics, tennis, ping-pong, track and field, and many other sports. Many professional team sports are dominated by men and women in their 20s and teens. Most of the talented 30-somethings are either burnt-out, drugged-out, or injured out of participating in the sports love of their lives. It is time to consider that the problem lies not in poor training techniques, but in the haphazard methods often applied to recovery.

There are four basic insufficiency factors involved in the body's ability to recover from training: insufficient sugar, insufficient salt, insufficient water, and insufficient rest and sleep. There is also one excess to consider—that of excess fat. When we understand how these five factors function and interact, we can use this knowledge to our best advantage in order to bring about the fastest recovery possible. It is well worth the effort. Athletes of all types will reap the healthy harvest of a speedy recovery and the ability to push their physical exertions to new and, perhaps, unimagined heights. Optimum recovery allows for more frequent training sessions, more intense training sessions, and a

> We know how to train far beyond our ability to recover. Isn't it time we put more attention on learning to recover?

sharper mind. Each of these factors results in fewer injuries, greater improvements in performance, and an overall increase in enjoyment in physical pursuits.

Chapter Three
SUGARS

Simple sugars in the form of glucose and/or fructose fuel every cell of the body. This sugar is found in the body as blood sugar and is converted into liver glycogen and muscle glycogen. Liver glycogen is mostly held in reserve as fuel for the brain. When we begin activity, the body first uses muscle glycogen to fuel the muscles, with minimal utilization of blood sugar. It takes approximately 2 hours of high-intensity aerobic activity (75–80+% VO2 max) to use up most of the available muscle glycogen. Toward the end of this period, blood sugar utilization begins to increase, and blood sugar levels start to fall. Within another hour or two of continued activity, depending upon the level of exertion, blood sugar levels must either be replenished through refueling or they will drop until activity cessation is forced.

Reestablishing blood sugar to normal levels and replenishing muscle glycogen are absolute requirements for efficient and effective recovery. This can be done most easily through the consumption of fresh, whole fruit shortly after exercise. Blood sugar levels respond to the consumption of fruit by rising at a moderate rate. Muscle glycogen supplies are somewhat slower in replenishing themselves, as muscles must rely upon the conversion of blood sugar to muscle glycogen. Muscle glycogen replenishment is accelerated during exercise, and at an ever-reducing rate back towards normal levels for about 2 hours after exercise is terminated, because the blood is flooded with an enzyme known as, "glycogenase." We produce this enzyme in quantities that double the body's ability to convert blood sugar into muscle glycogen. Thus, if sufficient blood sugar is available, it is possible to replenish muscle

> Sugar is "the spice of life" when it comes to athletic performance.

glycogen at double the normal rate during the 2-hour period immediately following exercise, thereby fostering a speedier recovery. This truly is a crucial time for athletes to eat properly, if they desire a speedy recovery.

If physical exertion is long enough or intense enough to seriously deplete the supply of muscle glycogen, it can take 24 hours or more to bring glycogen levels back to normal, even at optimal rates of replenishment. If the window of opportunity to replenish blood sugar and muscle glycogen stores directly following exercise is missed, or if the incorrect foods are eaten at those critical times, it can take more than twice as long to recover. Because of this, it is extremely important to supply sufficient fruit sugar before, during, and immediately after exercise, especially when it is long and/or intense. If this window is missed, training and recovery possibilities will be greatly reduced.

Bananas and grapes, along with a huge variety of other sweet fruits, contain sugars that allow for optimum speed of uptake. They have enough glucose along with their fructose to rate towards the top of all fruits in terms of their glycemic index. This index is, technically, "a system of evaluating the speed with which carbohydrates (sugars) are made available to the intestinal enzymes for hydrolysis and intestinal absorption." (Hydrolysis is the splitting of a compound, in this case, sugar, into fragments by the addition of water. The hydroxyl group is incorporated into one fragment and the hydrogen atom into another.) The glycemic index effectively measures how fast blood sugar concentrations rise after the consumption of specific quantities of carbohydrate from various foods.

Blended with enough water to provide adequate rehydration (sugars cannot be properly converted to glycogen without an ample stock of water in the body), bananas are one of the perfect foods for recovery after exercise. Serious athletes typically eat (or drink) 10 to 15 or more bananas for their postexercise meal.

Acid fruits high in sugar, such as pineapples, strawberries, tangerines, certain oranges, and some varieties of grapefruits, also provide the glucose and fructose necessary for quick replenishment of blood sugar and water needs. It is for this reason that bananas and oranges are usually provided during and after athletic competitions.

> Athletes commonly eat 1,500–2,000 calories for their post-workout meal. At 100 calories per large banana, eating 5–20 bananas after a training session makes all the sense in the world.

Other excellent postactivity fruit choices include, but are not limited to: figs, mangoes, peaches, nectarines, dates, apricots, plums, pears, and any other sweet fruit. Although lacking the fiber necessary for optimal health, freshly squeezed fruit juices also make excellent choices for speedy recovery after exercise. Even better are whole fresh fruits blended with water, or freshly squeezed citrus juice with the pulp included.

Cooked fruits provide the sugars necessary for recovery, but are lacking in enzymes and vitamins. The cooking process also results in the production of many mutagens and carcinogens, all of which are serious health destroyers. Hence, cooked fruits are not recommended. Fruit juices that have been pasteurized (heated to 161°F) also do not make acceptable substitutes for fresh juice, for the same reasons. In the heat of the pasteurization process, foods are stripped of many of their most valuable nutrients—enzymes, coenzymes, mineral, vitamins, antioxidants, and phytonutrients. These fragile substances begin to be destroyed at temperatures beginning as low 116°F. The heat of pasteurization also functions to denature proteins (this is how microbes are destroyed) and, thus, renders those proteins unavailable for human nutrition.

Chapter Four
MINERAL SALTS

Explaining chemistry is never as easy as it should be for a variety of reasons. Most important, perhaps, is the fact that chemistry is based on a system that is likely not accurate. The science of physics actually debunks most of the science of chemistry. But for lack of a better system, or a more accurate method of explaining the chemical nature of things, we use what we have. The other reason that chemistry is never easy to explain is because there are so many exceptions to almost every rule, so many complex variations on each theme, and so many overall possibilities. In each instance, to date, there is still a tremendous amount that we don't know or haven't yet tried or options that yield unpredictable results. That said, here are some basic definitions regarding salts and the minerals involved in their creation.

In nutrition, mineral salts are simple inorganic chemicals that are required, as nutrients, by living organisms. Important mineral salts include iron salts, magnesium salts (needed mainly by plants to make chlorophyll), and calcium salts. Mineral salts do not usually contain the element carbon and are, therefore, inorganic (organic compounds always contain carbon).

In chemistry, a salt has this relatively simple definition: the neutral compound formed by the union of an acid and a base.

There are also many definitions that are much more complex. For the purposes of this book, it makes sense to keep this section as simple, yet accurate, as possible while fully understanding that there are great complexities of science, many exceptions to every rule, and that each reader has specific interests and questions.

> "Ye are the salt of the earth."
> —Matt. 5:13

Mineral salts play a vital role in virtually every cellular function of the body. There are many mineral salts used in the body, each with its own specialized function. Salts take the form of electrolytes—positively and negatively charged ions. Electrolytes create electrical potential inside and outside of the cells. This potential is referred to as osmotic pressure. It is the osmotic pressure that encourages the movement of fluids through the cell's semipermeable membranes. Mineral salts make it possible for nutrients to flow into the cell and for waste products to flow out of the cell. Without osmotic pressure, there would be no life. When it comes to the body's mineral salts, a state of relative homeostasis is imperative. For the purposes of most athletic endeavors, it is important to focus primarily on just two minerals: sodium and potassium.

Sodium and potassium are two of the key minerals involved in electrolyte balance. Celery is one of the highest vegetable sources of sodium, although you will find sodium in all fruits and vegetables. Fruits and vegetables are also good sources of potassium, with bananas, tomatoes, dates, and avocados at the top of the list.

Inside the body, fluids of interest to the athlete are found primarily in two locations—inside the cells (intracellular) and outside the cells (extracellular). Sodium is the primary extracellular mineral, while potassium is the dominant intracellular mineral. Glucose "rides" into the cell on sodium, dissolved in water, when potassium and sodium enter the

> Salt tablets have been given to athletes for decades. The coaches and trainers didn't have a clue that they were actually harming their athletes. Salt consumption results in water retention, reduced perspiration, a reduced cooling effect, and kidney damage. Most likely, overdose of salt is the cause of football players dying on the practice field each summer.

cell. Cellular metabolic waste is carried out of the cell, also dissolved in water, effectively "hitched" to the sodium that leaves the cell. Too little or too much of either mineral in relationship to the other spells trouble for cellular function. This results in compromised performance, delays in recovery, and an overall reduction of health.

Excess sodium in the body is eliminated through the kidneys, though somewhat inefficiently (we can easily die of overdose from the amount of sodium found in just one ounce of table salt). Upon sufficient exertion, sodium is also lost via the sweat glands. Unusually great thirst, water retention, and extremely salty sweat are the first signs and symptoms of excessive sodium. Subsequent signs and symptoms include elevated blood pressure, edema, water weight gain, dry skin, extreme thirst, and eventual kidney failure. Excess sodium has an adverse effect on the body's electrolyte balance and water distribution, and a negative effect on athletic performance and recovery. Overall water weight goes down when salt consumption is reduced, yet at the same time, the total amount of water available to the body for metabolism goes up. The athlete, therefore, experiences less thirst, a lowered risk of dehydration, and an improved weight-to-strength ratio.

When there is excess sodium in the body, extracellular sodium is also lost via the perspiration that accompanies intense athletic endeavors. If too much sodium is lost, intracellular potassium is then pumped out of the cells to maintain the concentration gradient of the two electrolytes. With this loss of potassium, water also leaves the cells. As the cell membrane crenates, cellular function is compromised. The resulting muscle weakness is a common symptom of heat prostration.

A diet dominated by fruits and vegetables is extremely high in potassium. The kidneys are extremely well equipped to eliminate any excess potassium. There is no possibility of experiencing an overdose of potassium, regardless of diet, except in the case of kidney failure.

The body's need for homeostasis in the critical relationship between sodium and potassium is only one part of the story. The acid/alkaline balance of the body is critical as well. The acidic by-products of metabolism and those of physical activity must be neutralized by alkaline minerals. To support

Excess potassium = no problem
Excess sodium = big problem
Avoid all foods that have salt as an ingredient.

a proper acid/alkaline balance, foods with predominately alkaline minerals should make up the bulk of the daily caloric intake. All fresh fruits and vegetables fit this category.

Chapter Five

WATER

Our bodies, in good health, are composed of about 70 percent water, by weight. All body functions are dependent upon sufficient water. The body cannot absorb salts or convert sugars to glycogen without water. Water loss as low as 1 percent of total body weight is medically considered to represent a state of "mild dehydration." Should water loss go as high as just 5 percent of total body weight, it is considered cause for serious medical concern. In many sporting events, athletes are monitored closely for water loss, and are removed from competition should their loss equal or exceed the 5 percent mark for their own safety. Survival, not just successful competition, literally depends on this precious fluid. In order to thrive, in average conditions, the body requires a minimum of 1 gallon of water per day. This water can be obtained through a variety of sources.

Under normal circumstances, most of the body's water needs can be provided through the consumption of raw plant foods. Fresh fruits and vegetables provide the highest water-to-calorie ratio of any foods. The fact that they are highest in water of all foods is why the marketers of juicers use fruits and vegetables for their demonstrations. Starchy foods are commonly thought of as the best sources of carbohydrates (providing carbon and water, hence "hydrate"), and they do supply lots of carbon, but they certainly do not hydrate you. Try putting bread, rice, pasta, corn chips, or baked potatoes through a juicer and see how much water it releases.

Sun, wind, heat, high elevation, and strenuous exertion, however, all increase water loss dramatically, and sometimes imperceptibly. This makes it a sensible choice for active individuals to drink water upon rising and before mealtimes, if they have any doubt at all that they are getting enough water. It also makes extra good sense to avoid eating foods that provoke a feeling of thirst, especially foods that have salt added.

Eight to twelve glasses per day—That's how water-deficient the standard American diet is.

If you are planning a long or intense workout, especially if it will be in the sun and heat, or even at high elevation, you must be respectful of the fact that such a workout demands increased water consumption compared to normal. In such a situation, it is a good idea to drink water before beginning the exercise. Sweat during exertion acts as part of the body's complex cooling system. It functions effectively, however, only if the sweat evaporates from the skin, hair, and clothing. If the sweat actually drips off the body instead of evaporating, it loses its effectiveness as a cooling agent. It is prone to do so in conditions of high humidity, during extended bouts of extremely intense exertion, or when the environment is "close." In such cases, sufficient water must be consumed during the activity as well as after in order to insure that water losses are fully replenished.

Water must be given the highest consideration in the effort to recover as speedily as possible from strenuous activity. One early warning sign of dehydration is the cessation of perspiration despite ongoing heavy physical activity. Intense lethargy is an acute symptom, one that is often more powerful than an actual sensation of thirst. Often when a person is dehydrated, s/he will not actually be aware of the thirst. Typically, when water consumption is initiated, thirst usually returns and functions as an encouraging agent to consume even more water.

Scanty urination or dark yellow urine also indicates that the body is dehydrated. When in doubt, drink more water. It is better to drink too much than too little. A well-hydrated person will urinate an average of eight to 12 times during each 24-hour period. If urination frequency decreases to fewer than eight in a day, it is a sure signal that it is time to increase water consumption.

Not sure if you are thirsty? Try drinking some water. If it goes down easily, you likely are thirstier than you realize.

The bathroom scale is perhaps the best tool in evaluating water loss. A pint of water weighs 1 pound; a gallon weighs 8 pounds. Simply weigh in before and after physical activity. Based on the before and after weight, you will have a good idea of how much water to replenish after you train. That which does not come from your meal must come directly from water consumption. If in doubt, start by drinking water before beginning to consume food. This will make for better digestion than if you drink during the meal, and for faster uptake of the water.

Another option is to blend your post-workout fruit meal with sufficient water to meet your hydration needs. Monitoring your weight in this way will prove valuable in learning how much water loss accompanies various activities in different seasons of the year. With practice, you will be able to fine-tune your water consumption to perfectly match your losses so as to stay well hydrated at all times.

No commercial drink tastes as good as feeling well hydrated feels. Drink water to stay well hydrated. Dehydration is the most common reason that athletes experience limitations in their performance.

Chapter Six
Rest and Sleep

It is ideal to get sufficient rest and sleep before exercise so that the body does not feel tired as exercise begins. Perhaps the biggest misconception about exercise is that it adds energy. Quite to the contrary, exercise requires energy, and lots of it. It is true that exercise stimulates the body, and with this stimulation a wakefulness results that can be interpreted as a false sense of "energy." But when the stimulation wears off, the body is considerably more tired than when exercise began. Regular participation in challenging activities does increase one's overall fitness, however, and thereby accustoms the body to a greater daily output of energy.

The wisdom of the body ensures that a continuous stream of billions of bodily functions occur every moment and in exactly the correct manner. When the body gives us the sensations that we interpret as drowsiness, the best thing to do is rest or sleep. To exercise when tired goes against all logic. It's like eating when full or sunbathing on top of a sunburn. When the body asks for sleep, the answer should be in the affirmative. To deny the body its basic needs is to flirt with disaster. The real skill is in learning to listen to the body's cues and pay attention as it attempts to communicate its needs.

Cats are considered some of the most athletic of all animals. They rest and sleep 18+ hours per day. Many of the world's top athletes are known to rest and sleep 12+ hours per day. What makes you think you can reach the top of your athletic game on fewer than 8 hours of sleep per day?

How much sleep does a person need? The answer is simple. Enough.

How does one know when one has had enough sleep? At the instinctive level, this is simple too. It is a feeling, even more than a knowing. An infant knows without thinking when he or she is tired. The child *feels* it. When a baby has had enough rest and sleep, it's time to explore the world. Otherwise, it's time to drop off to sleep peacefully, without a care in the world.

Intellectually, however, this issue is more difficult for adults to figure out. Yet how does one know when it is time to eat or to drink or to use the bathroom? In truth, we rely on our feelings for these determinations, much more so than we rely upon the clock. Rest and sleep are no different. When we awake in the morning, if we feel fully alert, refreshed, rested, and awake, we've probably had enough sleep. If we feel like rolling out of bed to start the day rather than rolling over and going back to sleep, it is time to get up and get the day started. If we awake to the alarm clock drowsy and barely able to move, we've probably shorted ourselves on necessary sleep.

Sure, we can do it; we can get through the day. But mental clarity, physical prowess, and coordination on all levels will be compromised. Injury risk rises exponentially with sleep deprivation. The police estimate that almost three-quarters of all traffic accidents are at least somewhat related to driver drowsiness.

On a purely physical level, it's easy to get enough sleep. Just go to bed earlier, much earlier, and keep going to bed earlier, and sleep until the act of sleeping no longer seems pleasurable. When you start waking up refreshed and enthusiastically ready to start the day, you will have a clue as to just how early you actually need to go to bed. Getting enough sleep is grossly underrated and equally undervalued. If you want to see huge improvements in your athletic performance, experiment with getting loads more sleep than you currently allow yourself.

> Unless you are waking up simply bursting with energy, you are likely *not* getting enough sleep.

Securing proper rest is easily as important as getting sufficient sleep. There are many types of rest, including: physical, sensory, emotional, and physiological.

Physical rest is a relative issue; a matter of degrees. Slowing from a run to a walk, for example, gives us a relative rest, as does going from walking to standing, or standing to sitting. Complete physical rest is found by lying down in a comfortable position amid pleasant surroundings.

Sensory rest is achieved through closing the eyes and, if necessary, the ears, to all unpleasant sights and sounds and being surrounded by pleasant ones. Sensory rest includes many other aspects of the environment, including comfortable temperature and humidity, pleasing clothing and bedding, and an overall ambience in your surroundings that you would call agreeable. Sensory rest can only be achieved in surroundings where you feel safe and secure.

Emotional rest can be reached with practice and is represented by a feeling of calm and detached awareness, a condition of being completely at ease. To be in a state of emotional rest, one must be worry free to the degree of knowing that all is well.

Physiological rest is also a relative state. It can be achieved via the slowing of basal metabolism, which accompanies the sleeping state and is augmented during periods of reduced digestive demand.

To reduce the digestive demand, one can:

Eat more simply at each meal; that is, use fewer ingredients

Eat foods that are in accordance with our biological design

Eat within the limitations of your digestive capacity

Eat foods that require the least digestive effort

The deeper and more profound the rest, the faster the body rejuvenates itself and recovers from the exertions of the days gone by. Athletic performance is greatly enhanced when full recovery is garnered on a daily basis through utilization of

> Rest: it is so much more than just doing nothing.

sufficient rest and sleep. Rest is an activity, a valuable pastime, and should be respected as such.

Anytime the body is stressed and the physical, chemical, or emotional limits are pushed, it is important to allow extra time for rest and sleep. Less sleep is needed, on the other hand, when the body is on a maintenance program. In the same way as children that are growing, athletes that challenge themselves with physical stresses in order to improve strength, endurance, and/or speed invariably find that they need extra sleep, often as much as 20 to 40 percent more. The alternative—walking around tired for days and weeks on end—invites injury, amotivation, enervation, and sickness. Is it possible to sleep too much? No. If it's possible for a person to fall asleep, his or her body is signaling that sleep is what it needs.

Athletes who take care of themselves and remain well rested have the promise of many decades of participation in the fitness activities of their choosing, and a long and healthy life after competitive sports. For those who do not, there is the specter of crippling degenerative arthritis, heart disease, and cancer.

> If you'd rather roll over than roll out of bed, maybe you should. If you are using an alarm clock to wake yourself in the morning, you are systematically cutting short your sleep.

Anabolism is an ongoing process in the body. It is defined as any construction of complex structures from simpler ones by living cells. This is the process used by the body to create growth and repair. When we are at rest, anabolism progresses faster than when we are active. The reverse process, catabolism, is also ongoing in the body. Catabolism is defined as any deconstructive process by which complex substances are converted into more simple ones by living cells. Its fastest rate tends to be when we are active. The sum of all anabolic and catabolic activity within the body is referred to as metabolism. Homeostasis results when the total anabolic processes are in balance with the total catabolic processes.

When the volume of anabolic processes outpaces the amount of catabolic processes within the body, we experience growth. Growth represents a tremendous amount of work by the body and is accompanied by an increased need for sleep. Newborn babies show unprecedented growth rates and often sleep up to 20 hours per day. During the first year of life, most babies sleep about 16 hours per day, on average. By year two, sleep is reduced to about 14 hours, and by year three, down to about 12 hours per day. On days when children are extremely active, they invariably sleep for an extra hour or two. This increased need for sleep is due to the accelerated growth rates of young children. When a child goes through a growth spurt, his or her parents often first become aware of it by observing their child's increased need for sleep, whether the child is 6 or 16. Similarly, when athletes attempt to improve and grow, whether it be in muscular strength, muscular endurance, or in cardiopulmonary ability, they should make allowances for the fact that they will experience an increased need for sleep.

A balance of anabolism and catabolism represents metabolism in a homeostatic steady state. In this state, the body is maintaining itself, breaking down and building up at the same rate. In a healthy individual, this homeostatic state can be maintained throughout most of adult life. When sufficient sleep and/or nutrients are not supplied for the body to proceed with the normal anabolic flow, the rate of catabolism increases relative to the anabolic rate.

One theory states that this, in a cumulative fashion, is the cause of all aging. Physiological aging can be slowed, even reversed to some degree, by providing the body with good nutrition plus sufficient rest and sleep for sufficient anabolism to occur. In the simplest sense, we refer to this phenomenon as "healing," and also as "recovery." To the athlete, this translates directly into faster recovery, improved performance, a longer career, a lowered likelihood of injuries (especially those of overuse), better rehabilitation after injury, and a healthful and youthful life after competition.

> For any active person, sleep is easily as important as fitness training itself. In fact, sleep should be considered an integral part of any fitness training program.

29

Chapter Seven

PROTEIN

Biochemistry: any of numerous, highly varied organic molecules constituting a large portion of the mass of every life-form and necessary in the diet of all animals for the growth and repair of tissue. It is composed of 20 or more amino acids linked in a genetically controlled linear sequence into one or more long polypeptide chains, the final shape and other properties of each protein being determined by the side chains of the amino acids and their chemical attachments. Proteins include such specialized forms as collagen for supportive tissue, hormones to regulate physiological processes, hemoglobin for the transport of oxygen, antibodies for immune defense, and metabolic as well as digestive enzymes.

Protein in the human body is quite stable, almost totally recycled, and, therefore, needs replacing only in extremely minute quantities. The term "protein" comes from the Greek word, *proteios*, which means, "to take first place," or "of the first quality." Protein is the main functional constituent of every cell nucleus. Along with fat in animal cell membranes and various carbohydrates in plant cell walls, protein is integrated into the surrounding structure of every living cell. Its primary role in the body is to provide

> The question, "Where do you get your protein?" has been asked so many billions of times that by now you would think that someone would have actually figured out the answer.

the specific nutrient material necessary for growth and repair. The only bodily substances that do not normally contain protein are urine and bile, though proteins from other structures can generally even be found even here.

The body's need for protein has been so overstated, and with such frequency, that fear of protein deficiency has become a major issue that often discourages people from even considering dietary changes. This concern flies in the face of the fact that protein deficiency is so uncommon, worldwide, that there is no medical term for it.

A condition known as kwashiorkor was once thought to be a shortage of protein but is now known to be caused solely by a severe restriction in calories. The infirmity resulting from calorie restriction is properly referred to as marasmus. The word "kwashiorkor" has been dropped from the medical dictionary except in reference to the protein shortages that accompany the consumption of insufficient calories referred to as "marasmatic kwashiorkor."

Technically, it would seem to be conceivably possible to experience protein deficiency when on a calorie-sufficient diet composed solely of protein-free foods such as refined carbohydrates (alcohol, pure starch, or pure sugar) and/or refined fats (bottled oil). However, such persons would invariably become debilitated by any of a variety of other very severe health problems long before they had a chance to demonstrate the symptoms of what has proven to be no more than a phantom problem—protein deficiency.

The fact that most of the protein consumed by people today is cooked, hence, in an unusable form, highlights the human body's low need for protein. Protein is usable only when its amino acid chains are intact. Heat deranges the amino acid chains and causes the protein in foods to become "denatured," meaning they are no longer viable.

When people consume food that has been heated to 161°F or higher, the proteins in that substance become damaged and are no longer useful to the body. In fact, they are worse than "of no use" because heating proteins results in the formation of mutagens and carcinogens, both of which are extremely harmful. When we eat proteins that have been heated, the body identifies them as toxic substances that must be eliminated as quickly as possible. White blood cells function as the body's janitors. After eating cooked foods, white cell counts typically are raised to five or six times the normal low level in order to clean up the toxic mess.

The major concern in terms of protein consumption comes from eating too much, rather than not enough. An excess of protein has been linked to a great number of health concerns. These include but certainly are not limited to: obesity, cancer, heart disease, arthritis, kidney disease, and liver failure. Almost invariably, foods with a relatively high protein concentration have fat as their primary calorie source. Beef, pork, fowl, fish, and other animal flesh typically ranges from 35–65 percent of calories from protein, with the other 35–65 percent coming from fat. Dairy products, often touted as excellent protein sources, are actually very high in fat. The protein range for nuts and seeds is generally only in the low teens, as is the carbohydrate range, meaning that the remaining 70–80 percent of their calories comes from fat. This means that the overconsumption of protein invariably results in overconsumption of fat as well.

Protein's link to fat poses a problem for athletes beyond that of being overweight. Fat consumption is directly related to atherosclerosis and subsequent arteriosclerosis. These conditions result in a narrowing and hardening of the large- and medium-size arteries, which, in turn, reduce blood flow.

> White blood cells, the body's janitors, are the all-American cell, for we use them once and then throw them away. Constant and repeatedly high production of these cells, with no recovery, invariably leads to a crash in production. Such a crash leaves a person wide open to becoming extremely toxic, extremely rapidly, and is recognized as one of the primary markers for the condition known as AIDS.

> What is the big deal, anyway? Have you EVER met anyone who had a protein shortage? And by the way, there is no such thing as a *craving* for protein. Your body simply cannot crave protein.

33

Any condition that results in reduced blood flow directly hinders an athlete's performance. We will further discuss the problems linked to the overconsumption of fat in the chapter dedicated to fat.

Infants have the highest need for protein per calorie because they have the fastest rate of growth. Therefore, the protein density of mother's milk gives us a fairly accurate idea of the high-end of human protein requirements. Typically, mother's milk provides about 6 percent of its calories as protein. In their late teens or early twenties, human beings stop growing taller and their protein requirements decline accordingly. Beyond the age of about 30, even muscle growth does not contribute appreciably to the protein needs of men or women.

The repair of damaged cells, as occurs with cuts or bruises, and the replacement of worn-out cells, as found in the linings of the mouth, intestines, skin, and red and white blood cells, continues throughout life. Hair and nails continue to grow as well. As mentioned earlier, a level of protein intake so low that it disrupts these normal body functions is so rare as to be essentially unheard of and remains medically unnamed.

Contrary to popular belief, protein is not a good choice for the body as an energy source. In fact, it is typically the body's last choice for energy, after all available carbohydrates and fats have been used up.

Another myth is that eating protein builds muscle. Muscle building is an adaptive response to muscle usage, generated by the body when it perceives increases in gravitational resistance. It is possible, however, for protein intake to be low enough that muscle growth can be inhibited, but only when insufficient calories are consumed. For ath-

> Simply eating protein does not result in muscle growth. To gain muscle, you must persistently and consistently perform activities that demand muscular strength.

letes and others who wish to build muscle mass, a slightly higher consumption of protein may be necessary than for the general public. *This should be achieved by an increase in total food consumption, not by increasing the ratio of protein to fat or carbohydrate in the diet.*

Current research indicates that protein needs per calorie consumed do not rise as a function of increased physical activity or participation in athletic endeavors. Caloric needs do rise with increases in physical activity, however—double, triple, quadruple, and even up to 10 times those of a sedentary person—and the total amount of protein consumed by the athlete does rise accordingly.

Protein does not appear to play a critical role in athletic performance, either. Over an extended athletic contest such as bicycling in the Tour de France, it is possible that insufficient protein intake could hinder muscle growth. (Of course, such inadequate protein intake would only be possible via the two methods outlined earlier: insufficient calorie intake or the consumption of refined carbohydrates and refined fats.) But it still would not have an adverse effect on performance, per se. In addition, it is difficult to imagine that the huge quantities of calories consumed during such an event (Tour de France riders typically consume 10,000–14,000 calories per day while competing in that extreme event) would not provide more than enough protein.

The consumption of a variety of fruits and vegetables adequately meets human protein needs. Fruits typically offer single-digit protein, averaging around 6 percent of calories. The raw vegetables that most people are happy to consume in a salad contain an average of about 15 percent of calories from protein. Unlike the protein from cooked animal foods, the protein from raw fruits and vegetables is completely usable by the body. As a bonus, it comes with very low levels of saturated fats and essentially no cholesterol. Fruits and vegetables also provide us with plenty of fiber, an essential nutrient that is completely absent in animal fare.

> Bodybuilders gaze enviously at gorillas, in awe of their well-developed and powerful musculature. The gorillas nonchalantly continue munching on their whole, fresh, ripe, raw, organic fruits and vegetables.

Chapter Eight

FAT

Any of a large number of white or yellowish oily/greasy compounds that are widely found in plant and animal tissues serve mainly as a reserve source of fuel energy. In mammals, fat that is stored in connective tissue is known as adipose tissue. Adipose is deposited beneath the skin and around the internal organs, where it also protects and insulates against heat loss, concussive shock, and so forth. Fat also helps regulate cholesterol metabolism and is a precursor of prostaglandins.

Pure fats are colorless, odorless, and tasteless. Fat is a necessary, efficient source of energy that supplies humans with essential fatty acids, such as linoleic acid (omega 6) and linolenic acid (omega 3). An ounce of fat contains more than twice the stored fuel energy of an ounce of protein or carbohydrates. Fat takes considerable time to be digested in the stomach, resulting in the sensation of fullness after eating it. Various foods that are rich in fat can be used to alter the aroma and texture of foods. Fats are made chiefly of triglycerides, each molecule of which contains three fatty acids. These take the form of either solid or liquid esters of glycerol with fatty acids. Fat is used in the manufacture of soaps, paints, other protective

> Fat is extremely important to the athlete. It provides an essentially unlimited supply of fuel. The padding it offers helps prevent injuries. Fat even helps us to think properly. For all its importance, no one has ever asked me, "Where do you get your fat?" Could it be that that question simply isn't sexy enough?

coatings, and cooking. Fats are insoluble in water or cold alcohol but soluble in ether, chloroform, or benzene.

Fat fulfills many roles in the human body. It acts primarily as an insulator in a variety of fashions. Fat helps to protect the body from exposure to low temperatures and other forms of cold such as the combination of water and wind, reduces the trauma to organs and bones during any concussive force, and lines the outside of nerve tissue to ensure that the electrical currents of the nerve travel properly. Fat is integrated into the membrane of every cell, providing a double-sided moisture barrier that keeps intracellular contents inside the cell and extracellular contents outside of the cell. Fat is also essential for the proper functioning of the endocrine glands responsible for producing the body's hormones. In addition, fat serves as a backup fuel source to carbohydrates to help meet the body's fuel requirements.

Other noteworthy functions of fat include maintaining healthy skin, carrying the fat-soluble vitamins *A*, *D*, *E*, and *K*, and aiding in their absorption from the intestines. Fats also help the body use carbohydrates and *proteins* in a more efficient manner. It must be emphasized, however, that too much fat is as much a deterrent to good nutrition as is too little fat.

The greatest concern for athletes in relationship to fat lies in knowing how to choose "good" fats over "bad" fats, and knowing how much fat to consume. Good fats, essential to the health of every living cell, are referred to as "essential fatty acids." These fats are unsaturated, and when isolated, are found as liquids at room temperature. Bad fats are saturated, and either contain cholesterol or result in a rise in blood cholesterol when they are consumed. Saturated fats are a major factor in the development of heart disease; they are primarily found either in

> The sooner we give up on the idea that "more is better" when it comes to nutrition, and especially when it comes to fat, the sooner we have a chance of becoming a nation of healthy people and witnessing world record-shattering performances becoming the rule rather than the exception.

animal products or in prepared food products that have been partially or completely hydrogenated.

In the hydrogenation process, hydrogen is forced under pressure into the open links of a fat's carbon chain, saturating the fat with hydrogen. The result is a fat that is no longer chemically useful to the body, and is, in fact, harmful, since the body can only utilize fats that are not saturated. Human beings do not have the digestive power to break the chemical bonds of saturated fats. Because hydrogen cannot be removed from saturated fats to convert them back into unsaturated fats, the fats become chemically inert. This fat then circulates in the blood as globules that cannot be properly metabolized, all the while reducing the body's ability to uptake, transport, and deliver oxygen to the cells, clogging arteries, and directly increasing the risk of heart disease.

Below is a simple four-part test to help distinguish healthy fats from unhealthy fats.

First, we must determine whether or not the fat has been heated. Heated fats, even those that have not been hydrogenated, have lost their antioxidant qualities. Heated fats have been proven conclusively to be carcinogenic, contributing to the development of, or directly causing, cancer in humans. As well, heated fats usually have been "reduced," meaning that oxygen has been driven from them, causing an increased propensity towards rancidity. The consumption of rancid oil is a risk factor for a host of negative health conditions.

Second, we must determine whether the fat came from an animal or vegetable source. The fat from plants is invariably the healthier choice. Animal fat contains millions of times more cholesterol per bite than plant fat. Animal fats are rich in the adrenaline and stress factors secreted by the animal during its life. Consuming the animal's growth hormones has been linked with the growth of a wide assortment of cancers and other unwanted growths.

Third, we must consider the state of the fat. Is it solid or liquid at room temperature? Liquids will be better for us, for this indicates that the fat is at least primarily unsaturated.

Finally, we must ask, "Is this fat refined or in its whole form, complete with all its natural nutrients?" Whole foods invariably are more nutritious than refined foods, and this includes fats as well. Pure fat in a bottle cannot be considered to be a health food any more than pure sugar in a bag.

> Too much fat in the diet is easily as harmful to the athlete as is too much fat on the body.

We do not have a license to consume unlimited quantities of even the healthiest fats, however. Every time a person overeats on fats, s/he either undereats on carbohydrates or overeats on total calories, and therefore, diminishes health and performance capacity. Too much fat in the bloodstream limits oxygen transfer throughout the body. This fact, alone, should be enough to encourage anyone that is looking to improve athletic performance to reduce their fat intake. By overeating on fat, a person not only reduces the amount of glucose consumed but also inhibits the body's ability to uptake, transport, and deliver that glucose. This is a double whammy for the athlete.

A diet that is composed primarily of simple carbohydrates from whole, fresh, ripe, raw, organic fruits and vegetables, with less than 10 percent of calories from fat and less than 10 percent of calories from protein, will provide every health seeker with an optimum "caloronutrient" ratio for max-

> Heated fats should be treated like the poisons they are. Athletes who are serious about their performance need to shun them at all times.

imum health and performance. The fats found in fruits and vegetables also offer the exactly perfect ratio of Omega 3 to Omega 6, and in quantities that are ideal for human nutrition.

All fats should be eaten only in their unheated states, as found in fresh avocados and other fatty fruits, and also in raw nuts and seeds. Although the fat in these foods is primarily unsaturated, they do contain some saturated fat.

The percentage is quite low for fats found in fruits and vegetables, generally about 5 to 20 percent, compared to the 70 to

90+ percent saturated fat found in most animal products. The ratio of saturated to unsaturated fats is referred to as the S/P ratio (saturated fats to poly-unsaturated fats). Most books on nutrition are in agreement when they cite the ideal S/P ratio as 20/80, exactly the average ratio found in plants. The average S/P ratio in animal foods is 80/20, a relative magnitude that in every way diminishes human health and performance.

Plants foods also contain so little cholesterol that until very recently, it was impossible to discover any quantity at all. We now know that there is cholesterol in plants, but that there is more cholesterol in one hamburger than one would consume from an entire lifetime of eating a diet of vegan fare. Cholesterol is an alcohol lipid, or sterol, that is present in all animal fats. In the human body, cholesterol is an integral part of every membrane. The body itself produces its own cholesterol in precisely the amounts needed to perform all cholesterol-related functions. Any extra cholesterol consumed through our food is excessive and harmful to health and physical performance. It tends to build up on the arterial walls, hindering blood flow, reducing the transport of oxygen, glucose, and other nutrients across the vessel wall, and resulting in an overall rise in blood pressure.

Avocados, nuts, and seeds make an excellent addition to the evening meal once physical exertion is over for the day. They are delicious, digest well with acid fruits and most vegetables, make salads more satiating, and add the caloric density most athletes desire. The athlete who develops a taste for healthy fats while shunning the unhealthy ones will see a rapid improvement in his or her health and performance. This one change will provide dramatic results and make any dietary sacrifices seem insignificant by comparison.

Chapter Nine

STARCH

Starch *n.* [From starch stiff, cf. G. stärke, fr. Stark strong.] (Chem.) A widely diffused vegetable substance found especially in seeds, bulbs, and tubers, and extracted (as from potatoes, corn, rice, etc.) as a white, glistening, granular or powdery substance, without taste or smell, and giving a very peculiar creaking sound when rubbed between the fingers. It is used as a food, in the production of commercial grape sugar, for stiffening linen in laundries, in making paste, etc.

Webster's Revised Unabridged Dictionary

Scientists estimate that starches were introduced into the human diet relatively recently, approximately 10,000 or so years ago. They have played an increasingly greater role as a food source ever since. Americans today typically eat complex carbohydrate foods, also referred to as starches, at every meal and often in between meals, as well. Since the introduction of the "carbohydrate loading" craze in the 1960s, athletes have been encouraged to gain "lasting energy" by increasing the percentage of starches in their diet. In fact, there are so many reasons for completely omitting these foods from the human diet that it would take more than this chapter to delineate and explain all of them. The book, *Grain Damage*, touches on

> We love for our food to taste good, or better still, for our food to taste great. No one likes food that has no taste. Yet we all know that starches are tasteless, by definition. It is an undeniable fact that every dictionary confirms.

many of the health and performance problems brought on by these nutritionally lacking foods. Presented here are just a few of them:

1. Starchy foods, especially in their refined state, are exceptionally low in enzymes and in most vitamins. As evidenced in the term "complex carbohydrates," it is difficult for the body to break starches down into usable, simple carbohydrate components. Starches require cooking to even make them digestible, but even then, they remain unpalatable until flavor-enhancing agents are added. Needless to say, while heating starchy foods caramelizes their starches and makes them more digestible, the cooking simply takes a food that is already unfit for human consumption and destroys it nutritionally, leaving only emptier calories. Since these calories no longer contain their own vitamins and other micronutrients, they require outside sources of nutrients before they can be converted into usable fuel. This means that the body must drain its own reserves in order to make use of the calories in starchy foods. A reliance upon complex carbohydrate foods as a primary fuel source inevitably leads to nutritional bankruptcy and the eventual breakdown of health.

2. Starches contain an overabundance of acid-forming minerals, making them an unsatisfactory choice for the athlete. The waste products of metabolism from athletic activity all come in the form of acids that must be eliminated from the body in order for the body to recover. The introduction of several daily doses of acidic minerals from starchy foods works directly against the body's self-interest. A hugely valuable step in supporting the body in maintaining an alkaline blood pH level is the elimination of starches from the diet. In health, the pH of the blood—a measurement of alkalinity and acidity—always remains on the alkaline side of neutral at about 7.4. If it varies by even two-tenths

of a point, health is at risk. A blood pH level of 7.0, which is neutral, is considered a severe medical emergency, and many people have died from hypo-alkalinity of the blood before the pH dropped even this low. While some athletes have been monitored with a blood pH as low

> Did you ever stop to wonder who it was that promoted the concept that the primary ingredient of wallpaper paste would make the ideal food for athletes?

as 6.9 during intense exercise, this definitely is not within the parameters of healthy performance training, nor is such an extremely low pH to be recommended. The blood pH of these athletes return to 7.4 within an extremely short time after exercise is terminated.

3. There is no model in nature for human grain consumption. Our anthropoid primate cousins—the chimpanzees, gorillas, orangutans, bonobos, and mandrills—consume no grains whatsoever. All animals, with the exception of humans and the animals they have domesticated, consume only the foods to which they are biologically adapted. And none of them, with the exception of a few varieties of birds and insects, consume grains at all. Wild animals consume all of their food in its whole, raw state. Would you ever even consider eating raw starch? If you do, you will likely only do it one time.

   If it were physiologically sound for us to eat starches, nature would dictate that we eat them in their whole, raw state. In this condition, however, we find that starches are not only unpalatable, but that they are also indigestible.

4. The narcotic, opium, is known for its addictive and sedating qualities. Chemists have discovered fifteen separate opiates in wheat. These are molecular structures similar enough to opium to cause an opiumlike response by the body. Athletes look for high-energy foods, not foods that leave them feeling drugged and addicted. For this reason,

if no other, starches should be off the training table of anyone serious about their fitness and health.

5. The consumption of starch is linked to hundreds of health issues, the most notable being congestion. For the athlete, being able to breath is critical. The gluten in most starchy foods is mucus-forming. The human body responds to its consumption by generating mucus both as a form of protection and to carry the gluten out of the system. A clogged up nose is not the only affliction the athlete suffers when eating starches, however. The ear canals, which play a vital role in balance and proprioception, tend to become clogged with mucus as well. Eating starchy foods result in a loss of balance, proprioception, co-ordination, and fine motor control.

> The addict's life revolves around the next "fix." The life of an athlete revolves around the next competition. What does the starch-addicted athlete live for—the next competition or the next meal?

6. Starches are promoted for athletes because of their supposed slow release of energy. The assumption made is that when we eat starches, we get a timed release of this fuel source. The assumption is incorrect. The starches take considerable time to be digested, and during that time, they give nothing. Rather, they demand fuel and energy in order to be digested. When they finally are digested, the entire load of fuel from that starch meal becomes available in a relatively short period of time, often overloading the system with sugar and resulting in an extreme drop in energy. Have you ever experienced an uncontrollable lull at ten in the morning or at three in the afternoon?

Athletes need an immediate and rapid release of energy in order to perform, especially if they wish to outperform the competition. A slow release means that they must wait hours to benefit from the foods they have eaten. The slow digestion of starch requires much more energy than the rapid digestion of the simple carbohydrates found in fruit and results in additional loss of energy to the digestion process. All in all, you get more carbohydrate benefit, and get it much more rapidly, by consuming your calories from a meal of sweet-tasting fruit rather than from tasteless starch.

7. Few but the most stoic people eat their starchy foods in a completely bland form. Starches taste so plain that usually copious quantities of fat or simple carbs are added to them to enhance the texture and the flavor. Other substances are also used to give flavor to starchy foods because they are so bland. Supposedly to improve the taste of starchy foods, sugar, salt, pepper, mustard, spices—in fact, an entire array of irritants and stimulants—are added. None of these substances are helpful in terms of athletic performance. The athlete who wants to take the next step in nutrition must leave the starches behind and move forward into the world of fruits. Vegetables, nuts, and seeds certainly play a role in the diet, but fruit, not starches, must predominate if an athlete wishes to attain maximum levels of performance.

All the calories that we eat, at least all of those that we digest and absorb, are converted into simple sugar, with the exception of the excess, which is converted into fat to be stored. It makes far more sense, nutritionally and energetically, to eat those simple sugars in their most wholesome form, directly from fruit, than it does to ask the body to convert proteins, fats, or complex carbohydrates into simple sugars.

Try eating a mouthful of cornstarch, straight from the box. You will see why Mary Poppins didn't sing, "Just a spoon full of cornstarch helps the medicine go down."

Chapter Ten
VITAMINS

Vitamins are defined as "organic substances, found in very small amounts in various foods, that are necessary for normal metabolic function of the species and provided only through the creature's diet." These substances are chemically unrelated to one another and may be water-soluble or fat-soluble. Interestingly, what qualifies as a vitamin or nutrient to one creature may not be a vitamin for another. For example, humans must provide for their vitamin C needs through their diets, whereas dogs can synthesize their own. Hence, vitamin C is not considered a vitamin for a dog.

One of the greatest concerns people have about their nutrition is whether or not they are ingesting enough vitamins without getting too much. When the diet is composed of a variety of whole, fresh, ripe, raw, organic fruits and vegetables, plus small quantities of optional nuts and seeds, there is the guarantee of sufficient intake of vitamins without any possibility of an overdose.

Vitamins serve many essential roles in human health. Without them, or without sufficient quantities of them, diseases of vitamin deficiency, such as scurvy, rickets, beriberi, and pellagra, develop. There are 15 known vitamins. Eleven of them are water-soluble and four of which—vitamins A, D, E, and K—are fat-soluble. It is possible, through the use of supplements, to consume toxic levels of the fat-soluble vitamins. Overdoses lead to serious illnesses and can result in death. The rest of the known vitamins are water-soluble and excreted through the urine when excessive quantities are ingested or when high concentrations of these vitamins build up in the bloodstream. This makes the possibility of water-soluble vitamin toxicity rather unlikely.

> In our pill-popping nation, it is sadly funny that the vast majority of people are worried about the unlikely event of health issues developing from vitamin deficiency, while almost none are concerned about the very real likelihood of health issues developing as a result of vitamin excess.

Researchers are constantly learning and understanding more about the nature and function of vitamins. It has been found that two groups of compounds are chemically related to vitamins. These are precursors known as pro-vitamins and antagonists known as analogs. Pro-vitamins are substances that have no vitamin activity until the body converts them into the usable form of the vitamin. Sometimes the conversion requires other factors, such as sunlight, which must shine directly on the skin in order for the body to convert 7-dehydrocholesterol into vitamin D.

Analogs usually are chemically related to the biologically active vitamins, although not necessarily so. The analog will actually be substituted into the cell, or the uptake site, in place of the true vitamin, thereby blocking the vitamin from entering and, thus, preventing proper function. The effect is akin to putting the wrong key in a lock, breaking it off, and being unable to remove it. For example, an analog for B-12 is generated when the B-12 on plant matter is dehydrated. This B-12 analog uses the same receptor sites as the true B-12 and, therefore, limits the body's ability to uptake B-12.

Other substances, classified as anti-vitamins, are important when discussing vitamins. These substances function by actually damaging or destroying active vitamins, rendering them worthless. It is possible to literally strip oneself until bankrupt of a given vitamin through long-term exposure to its anti-vitamin. Fortunately, anti-vitamins of this sort are not

> By eating only raw fruits, vegetables, nuts, and seeds, it is difficult, if not impossible, to develop a vitamin deficiency.

found in any foods to which we are biologically adapted. Predominantly, they are found in toxins such as cigarette smoke, alcohol, and coffee. It is interesting and important to note that they have also been discovered in eggs and flesh foods of all varieties.

For all we have learned about vitamins, it has never been demonstrated that any excess amount of any vitamin has a positive effect on athletic performance. It has been clearly shown, however, that mega doses (referred to in some literature as an "orthomolecular dose," or "orthomolecular medicine") of some vitamins will have a predictably negative impact on athletic performance and personal health. Beyond the normal daily requirements, sufficient vitamin intake should not be a concern.

Many vitamins are destroyed by exposure to temperatures above 130°F, however, and, as food is our only natural source of vitamins, they cannot be reconstructed within our body from their component parts. Once damaged by heat, the nutrient material that once was a vitamin is, at best, useless to the body. At worst, it is treated as a foreign substance to be contained and eliminated, serving as another drain on the body's energy reserves and limiting athletic performance.

To maximize nutrition and minimize the negative effects of toxic matter upon the body, the athlete does well to design his or her diet to include as much whole, fresh, ripe, raw, organic fruits and vegetables as possible. If s/he wishes to include nuts and seeds, these should be consumed in relatively small quantities that rarely, if ever, exceed 5 percent of the total calorie intake for the day.

Fruits and vegetables are the most nutritious of all foods. This means, effectively, that their nutrient content most closely mimics human nutritional needs. Eating a diet predominated by fruits and vegetables, or one that is made up exclusively of fruits and vegetables, should, therefore, only instill confidence in the consumer. Such a diet should be the cause of virtually no doubts or fears about nutrition, performance, or overall health.

Chapter Eleven
ENZYMES

Enzyme (ĕn'zīm)—Any of numerous proteins produced in living cells that accelerate or catalyze the metabolic processes of an organism. Enzymes are usually very selective in the molecules that they act upon, called substrates, often reacting with only a single substrate. The substrate binds to the enzyme at a location called the active site just before the reaction catalyzed by the enzyme takes place. Enzymes can speed up chemical reactions by up to a millionfold, but only function within a narrow temperature and pH range, outside of which they can lose their structure and become denatured. Enzymes are involved in such processes as the breaking down of the large protein, starch, and fat molecules in food into smaller molecules during digestion, the joining together of nucleotides into strands of DNA, and the addition of a phosphate group to ADP to form ATP. The names of enzymes usually end in the suffix -ase.

The American Heritage Science Dictionary

Enzymes are the organic chemistry version of the catalysts we know from physical chemistry. They perform thousands of specialized functions within the human body, allowing various processes to begin while not involving themselves in the actual process itself. There are over 500 enzymes in each cell that are involved solely in the final stages of assimilation of nutrients—either in the release of energy or in the incorporation of nutrient material into body structure. Some enzymes work alone, while others require the aid of coenzymes to initiate their actions.

Fresh fruits, vegetables, nuts, and seeds contain within themselves all the enzymes necessary for completing their own ripening processes. In the case of fruit, the ripening process is actually similar to what we call digestion. Complex carbohydrate molecules are broken down into simple sugar molecules and water. For this reason, unripe fruit with its complex carbohydrates does not taste as sweet as its ripe counterparts with simple carbohydrates. In legumes, the process moves in the opposite direction, with simple sugars being converted to complex carbohydrates as the legume matures. This process is called "setting starch" and explains why very young legumes taste sweet, while fully mature ones taste starchy. All ripening processes are controlled by the influence of enzymes.

> Enzymes are much like your own front door key. The key makes it possible for you to enter your home by letting you change the lock's position, but the key itself remains unchanged before, during, and even after the locking (or unlocking) processes are completed.

The enzymes involved in the ripening of fruit should not be confused with the enzymes utilized by the body to digest foods. If, in fact, they were one and the same, foods would digest themselves on your kitchen counter. Imagine reaching into your cupboard for a jar of almonds, only to find that they had digested themselves into a mass of some jelly-like goo. There are over 20,000 enzymes produced by the body in order to keep our physiology running properly. A mere 20 of those are directly involved in the digestion of carbohydrates, proteins, and fats. Your body manufactures all of these enzymes, as necessary, for your entire lifetime, much like it manufactures tears, saliva, or perspiration.

> Think big; think "whole foods" and you will remain invincible. When you fall for the trap of eating for the micronutrients in foods rather than for the foods themselves, you have lost the plot. At that point, you have become vulnerable.

Enzymes are the most heat-sensitive of all nutrient substances. Some begin to be inactivated (lose functionality) at temperatures as low as only 116°F. Every form of cooking destroys the enzymes in food, along with the other protein structures in the food. Once the proteins in food are damaged, including the specific proteins in enzymes, there are no bodily processes that can repair them. They will be recognized by the body as useless and potentially dangerous foreign proteins and will be contained and eliminated. Thus, the consumption of cooked food invariably results in a steady drain on the body's protein and nutrient reserves since there are nutrients constantly being used by the body but not being resupplied by the food consumed.

Whether foods are cooked or not, the body requires a massive number of enzymes to complete the processes of digestion (in the intestines), absorption (into the bloodstream, into the lymphatic system, and, eventually, into the cell), and utilization (by the cell). These specific enzymes are generated from the body's protein and nutrient reserves. The body always manufactures a wide assortment of enzymes as a response to the consumption of food. If the food consumed is cooked, with the proteins and other nutrients damaged, the result will be an ever-growing deficit that can only lead to nutritional bankruptcy.

Long before a state of total nutritional bankruptcy immobilizes the body, many bodily processes are adversely affected by the growing inability to manufacture the necessary enzymes. Clinical signs and subclinical symptoms associated with the lack of ability to produce a specific enzyme often are evidenced by unhealthful accumulations of debris and toxins in the tissue or blood. In every such case, low levels of enzymes result in performance deficits. Much of the

> Key in to that which is most important. Unlock the door that leads to high-level performance. The enzymes in foods are valuable nutrients. The enzymes produced by the body are essential for life. The enzymes sold as supplements are simply pills—emperor's clothing, and nothing more.

fine-tuning that results from improvements in nutrition is subclinical, meaning that it will not necessarily yield overt, demonstrable results. Yet the lack of important nutrients can only lead to a drop in performance abilities, and remedying the situation can only be viewed as a positive step. As with all aspects of self-care, eating healthfully has no contraindications.

Chapter Twelve
WEIGHT CONTROL

Weight control is a major issue for athletes. Surprisingly, there are almost as many athletes who want to gain weight as there are those wish to lose weight. Both losing and gaining weight are relatively simple if one understands the physiology behind the process. The following information works equally well for everyone, even those who simply wish to maintain their weight.

The overfat athlete has obvious problems. Excess body fat hinders speed, agility, flexibility, and practically every other aspect of performance. Yet, it is an exceptionally slow process for an athlete to lose fat through additional exercise. Athletes already live extremely active lives, and it is difficult for them to add even more activity into their days. In addition, activity itself does not burn off huge amounts of calories. Running an extra mile per day barely adds up to a loss of ten pounds in an entire year.

The simplest way to lose the excess body fat is to eat foods that are lower in calories per bite than the foods you currently eat. For example, by increasing the amount of raw vegetables consumed, one can make a large difference in the total calorie intake for a day.

A head of lettuce about the size of a double or triple cheeseburger packs 24 calories while the cheeseburger offers up 800–1,200, depending upon the vendor. The low calorie-per-bite foods also take longer to

> When it comes to weight loss, it is important to be extremely clear: Is the program you are following causing you to lose muscle, fat, or water?

chew than processed foods, because fiber requires chewing, and it is the fiber that is typically removed from processed foods. Vegetables typically take longer to eat than processed foods, giving the consumer more of a chance to feel full before actually overeating.

Fruits provide the second-lowest calories-per-bite ratio of all the food groups, and they are filled with a satiating sweetness. This sweetness is combined with lots of fiber, so that rises in blood sugar are moderated. Nonetheless, the sugar in fruit serves as a valuable factor that successfully reduces the appetite, often completely. The low calorie intake and the satiating quality of fruit makes it an excellent choice, along with vegetables, for those who want to lower their total body fat percentage by losing body fat.

Most Americans are undermuscled and overfat. Those who manage to lose excess fat, or who never have gained it in the first place, generally are still undermuscled and tend to appear "painfully thin." The remedy for this situation is straightforward. One must gain muscle. Muscle is dense, heavy tissue. When muscles grow, they do not increase in the number of muscle fibers but in the number and size of the mitochondria, the organelles inside the muscle fibers that are responsible for generating energy. It is quite possible to gain a pound of muscle weight per month through the institution of a well-designed resistance program.

There are many styles and philosophies of weight training, and most of them work sufficiently well. Results vary according to the frequency, intensity, and duration of training, along with the degree of recovery achieved. Generally, lower repetitions with heavier weights will result in greater muscle gain than will a high number of repetitions with lower weights. A muscle-gaining program, like any other conditioning work, should begin gradually and progress steadily.

If you participate in the same workout day after day, you are likely maintaining your fitness, but not making any training gains. In order to train, you must either perform activities that you are not used to, or perform those that you are used to in ways that you are not used to doing them.

It should be approached consistently and persistently, and viewed with long-term as well as short-term goals. The trick to growing muscle, if, indeed, there is a trick, is to make certain that one is using the exercise time for training, rather than using it solely for maintaining one's fitness.

The person who trains intensely will feel a need to eat more calories per day than the person who is sedentary. This poses no problem. Caloric density can best be achieved through the consumption of nuts, seeds, avocados, and other fatty fruits. The athlete wishing to gain muscle mass will also find a rich source of amino acids (required to increase the size and number of mitochondria within the muscle fiber) in nuts and seeds. Avocados are primarily a source of fat and do not carry as high a percentage of protein as do nuts and seeds. That said, it is in our best health interests to never allow the ratio of carbohydrate to protein to fat to fall below 80 percent of calories from carbohydrates, or above 10 percent of calories from protein or from fats, as an average in the diet. The active individual will invariably consume a greater number of calories overall, but the 80/10/10 ratio still must be respected, or predictable health and performance decline will ensue.

Many combinations of fat loss and muscle gain, or vice versa, are possible. A person losing two pounds of fat but gaining two pounds of muscle shows no total weight change. It is possible to gain two pounds of fat and lose two pounds of muscle, again showing no net gain or loss of weight. The use of a bioimpedance monitor, or calipers, to measure total body fat percentage is, therefore, extremely useful. With such monitoring tools, the athlete can keep a very accurate track of his/her body fat percentage. This information sheds valuable light on any weight fluctuation shown on the scale, or any lack thereof.

Achieving and maintaining a goal weight is a worthy aim and necessary in

> An overly fat person cannot be completely healthy. Excess fat inhibits all vital functions. Your overall health, like your overall fitness, can only be as good as its weakest link.

order to consistently perform at peak. Before doing so, however, a realistic first step is to bring overall body fat to the percentage that is desired. Then, if weight gain is still desired, the obvious answer is to gain muscle mass. Using a combination of a scale and a body fat monitoring device, the athlete takes all the guesswork out of weight management. Far too many athletes fool themselves into thinking that much of their weight is muscle, when, in reality, it is excess fat.

Athletes who have managed the feat of stabilizing their weight can move on to other productive aspects of training. A balanced approach to cardiopulmonary, muscular strength, muscular endurance, flexibility, and neurological training will provide maintenance levels of each without resulting in excessive muscle growth. The same is true for the diet, with "balance" being the key word. A balanced diet is one composed of whole, fresh, ripe, raw, organic fruits, vegetables, nuts, and seeds, with fruits providing roughly 90 percent of the overall calorie intake. When any active person replaces their usual Westernized diet, with its unbalanced formula predominated by cooked proteins and starches, it will be the beginning of true lifelong health and weight control.

If eating well were easy, everyone would do it. In fact, eating healthfully and being healthy is far easier than eating poorly and being sick as a result. Athletes that try this approach to eating invariably stick with it, even after their competitive careers end, because the results are more than worth any work that they may have to put into following the 80/10/10 program. The same is true for fitness. If fitness training regularly for a lifetime were easy, everyone would be fit. But again, in fact, a lifetime of fitness is far easier to endure than a lifetime of infirmity, and well worth the effort.

> We learn how to eat well by eating well. It gets easier with practice, like everything does. Maintaining your optimum weight for a lifetime is the goal, and this is achieved through steadily eating well, day in and day out. Drastic approaches to weight management teach you nothing about weight maintenance, and only lead to frustration.

Chapter Thirteen

STIMULANTS

Reliance upon stimulants is epidemic in the world of sports. It is important to know, however, that stimulants only give a short-lasting spurt of false energy because the net effect of their use is that they actually rob the body of energy. It is imperative to understand what stimulants are and how the energy that appears to come from them is used only to ameliorate their chemical effects. Stimulants are not the "sources" of energy for which we give them credit. They are toxic, at every dose. Quite simply, stimulants result in a bodily-generated increase in the activity of the sympathetic nervous system, the central nervous system, or, in the case of certain stimulants, both systems.

The body's response to the consumption of a stimulant is to release some of its stored energy reserves in order to more rapidly eliminate the stimulant from the body. This is done, in the case of stimulants, via the increased action of various components of the nervous system. Coffee, cigarettes, tea, cola, refined sugars, chocolate, spices, meat, amphetamine-type drugs, and many other substances are all stimulants that actually increase the body's workload and drain its vital reserves of energy. Over 80 percent of Americans consume caffeine on a daily basis, and numbers in the low 90 percent are reported for the occasional use of this stimulating substance

The only physiological mechanism for accumulating energy in the human body is sleep. We learn this simple lesson every night of our lives, yet somehow, most people manage to overlook it.

A healthy person goes to bed at about the time their energy wanes and wakes in the morning with energy restored for another day. The person who wakes up and still feels tired simply needs more sleep. The quantity of sleep required, in terms of hours, is not based upon the clock, but upon the body's needs. Some nights, more is required, and some nights, less. The more physically active we are, the more sleep that is typically required. Athletes are notorious for sleeping long hours.

How, then, is this energy properly delivered to the various tasks of the day? The answer is certainly not through the use of stimulants. Although their consumption results in a release of energy, it invariably ends up adding to the energy and sleep needs of the day. The ability to output energy at greater levels actually comes through exercise. It comes with the conditioning that involves vigorous overload and proper recovery. Constructive conditioning includes muscle training that is geared toward putting out more energy than usual, in the same amount of time, and to exerting as usual, but for a longer duration than customary. Coupled with sufficient recovery, such a training program eventually translates into the ability to put out more energy per unit of time for more units of time. This is referred to as the "training effect."

Energy is measured in units called calories, which are, technically, units of heat. When the number of calories is given for a food, it actually refers to the number of potential heat units the body can liberate from that food. This means that a calorie measures not

> Feeling low on energy, but not sure what to do about it? Most people just check to see what time it is. If it is daytime, they take a stimulant of some sort, or a combination of them, such as a chocolate pastry and a cup of coffee. If it is evening, they resort to watching a stimulating movie, or they eat some sweets. Finally, if it is somewhat past bedtime, they give in and go to sleep. In reality, it is the sleep that results in the energy required to face the upcoming day. The stimulant use was an ineffective attempt to make up for getting insufficient amounts of sleep, and only serves to make matters worse.

kinetic energy but potential energy. In other words, references to calories do not measure the energy in a food, but the quantity of fuel provided by the food for producing energy.

According to this system of measurement, the potential energy supplied by a cup of coffee can be measured by counting the number of calories in the cup of coffee. How many calories are there in a cup of black coffee? Zero. How much potential energy does it supply? Zero. Therefore, all of the energy demonstrated by the body as a response to the stimulation from the chemicals in the coffee was already in storage in the body. The body released some of its precious stored energy to deal with the effects of the caffeine and the other chemicals in the coffee. The coffee supplied nothing back except toxins. It certainly did not supply more fuel for the body to build more energy since the calorie count was zero. The act of drinking a cup of coffee actually produces a net requirement for more sleep than usual. Coffee and other stimulants are not energy suppliers for the body; they are energy drainers of the highest type.

> Sleeping is the only effective and healthful way to accumulate energy in the body. In the same way that a muscle requires deep and full relaxation in order to demonstrate complete and efficient contractions, we need sufficient hours of restful sleep in order to demonstrate our fullest vigor when awake.

Not only is the physical performance of an athlete hindered when s/he is exhausted, but also the risk of injury increases dramatically. The tired athlete cannot think clearly, even to the point of not being aware that s/he is not thinking clearly. In the high-performance world of competitive sports, this makes for a dangerous situation. Undue risks may be taken, poor judgment is more often shown, and timing is off when the athlete is tired. The use of stimulants only worsens this situation in two ways.

First, the athlete is fooled into thinking that s/he is functioning properly when, in fact, this is not the case. All functions are impaired when we are tired.

Second, the use of stimulants may result in increased gross muscle abilities, but it does so at the loss of fine motor control. Ball-handling skills, hand-eye coordination, "touch" skills, and all other delicate movements' fine control is seriously compromised with stimulant usage.

> Like the abilities "gained" from the use of any drug, the energy "gained" from the use of a stimulant is strictly illusory.

All aspects of anabolism are hampered due to stimulant usage. All other things being equal, recovery is much slower for a tired athlete than for a well rested one. If the second worst thing an athlete can do is to obtain insufficient sleep, then the worst is to begin using stimulants, or to continue to use them. The amount of stimulation one person will experience from a substance cannot be predetermined, but we do know that what is a stimulant for one person is a stimulant for another. We also know that the body wears down from stimulant use, vital reserves become drained, that the ability to respond will become reduced as a result of increased tiredness, and that the body will adapt over time to a stimulant.

To overcome these factors, athletes must use not only more of the same stimulating substances, but they typically turn to stronger substances as well. The gamble is huge for the athlete that relies on stimulants in order to be able to perform. Take too much of the stimulant and run the risk of injury plus the risk of being banned from competition. Take too little and give a subpar performance.

When the stimulant in question is a "legal drug," the guessing game becomes even more complicated than we might suspect. Caffeine is found in many substances other than coffee. The athlete might drink two and a half cups of coffee, an allowable amount according to international standards for sports, and assume that s/he is safe to compete. However, the amount of caffeine found in some over-the-counter cold remedy, a chocolate bar, a soft drink, or some other "hidden" source could easily put the unsuspecting athlete over the allowable limit. If not penalized by the governing body of their sport for going over the limit on stimulant consumption, unknowingly taking large quantities of a stimulant will negatively effect fine motor control and will likely result in reduced athletic performance overall.

> This is your body.
> This is your body on stimulants.

If we truly wish to know which athlete is the most talented, the best prepared, the best able to rise to the pressures of competition, there is only one sane option. Ban all substances not naturally found in the body or in our food, and ban higher-than-normal—concentrations of all naturally occurring substances.

Of course, there is another option. If we want to watch a bunch of drug-crazed people risking life and limb in order to give superhuman performances in their efforts to win, then all substances should be legalized. Let the records fail and the athletes' health fail.

We certainly are not demonstrating concern for the health of the athletes by the policies we currently use. Perhaps it is time to allow athletes to do whatever they wish. After all, they are grown-ups, aren't they? Who cares if they set the model for younger athletes to follow? Should we be concerned if the injury rate soars? If this sounds like lunacy, it is. But then, so is the current drug policy. The only safe and sane drug policy is the zero drug policy.

With sufficient sleep, stimulant use becomes unnecessary, redundant, and downright ridiculous. Without enough sleep, the athlete's life is terribly draining. The tired athlete performs poorly. Health, happiness, energy, and motivation all dissipate quickly. The injury rate skyrockets. These are the initial markers that indicate that the athlete is being robbed of precious vitality. The catabolic aging process speeds along almost completely unchecked by recovery's anabolic counterbalance. Careers rush by, foreshortened by a simple lack of sleep. For an athlete to produce truly high-quality performances on a regular basis over a long and lasting career, s/he must rely on

> Oh where, oh where has my energy gone? Oh where, oh where can it be? With my sleep cut short and my workout long, Oh where, oh where can it be?

sleep, not on stimulants, for energy production. This sane and healthy approach will result in athletes who are consistently more capable of performing at their peak, more dynamic and exciting to watch, and who will be with us for a longer time.

Chapter Fourteen

FOOD COMBINING

For an athlete to perform at maximum efficiency, the body must direct as much blood as possible to the muscles. Most athletes achieve this delivery of blood through their mental and physical training. If an athlete is not aware of correct food combining strategies, however, he or she misses out. This important technique frees up blood, hence, fuel and oxygen, from the digestive process so that it can be sent to the body's musculature.

The optimum meal for the speediest and easiest digestion is a simple one, usually made up of only one ingredient. It is possible, however, to digest a more complex combination of foods with relative ease. This is accomplished by learning how to combine foods so that their digestion requires as little blood flowing to the digestive system for as short a period of time as possible.

Each person carries a limited supply of blood. The volume varies with the size of the person, but it is sufficiently accurate for our purposes to say that the average person carries approximately 11–12 pints of blood. There is not enough total blood volume to service all parts of the body at the same time, at least not while they are all functioning fully. Children are taught not to go swimming immediately after eating for good reason. After a meal, large quantities of blood flow automatically to the digestive system. If large quantities of blood are demanded by

> It isn't enough for an athlete to simply eat great food. S/he must also digest, absorb, assimilate, and eliminate it optimally.

the muscles while the digestive tract is functioning at full pace, there will simply not be enough blood to do both jobs.

With insufficient blood supply to the muscles, there is the distinct possibility of muscle cramping, a dangerous occurrence for swimmers in deep water. It is also very likely that even if muscle cramps don't ensue, that the digestive system will not get all the blood it requires, and that the digestive processes will be delayed. This will lead to the food in the intestines going bad rather than digesting, resulting in fermenting carbohydrates, putrefying proteins, and fats going rancid.

There is another classic situation that demonstrates the value of food combining. An old proverb says, "Blood goes either to the brain or to the stomach." This proverb is very well respected. In many countries, it is common to do business over a meal, but the smart businessmen talk first and eat later, while they encourage their clients to eat first and talk later. The truth of this old saying can be observed in most households after every holiday meal, where the family falls asleep while watching the television set.

A large meal, particularly one that is difficult to digest, can require upwards of 50 percent of the total blood supply to the organs of digestion. This leaves insufficient amounts for other functions, and certainly an insufficient quantity to perform vigorous exercise. So, the blood supply to the muscles is minimized for a period of time, while blood supply to the organs of digestion is maximized. For this reason, people feel lethargic after a large meal. With most of the blood carrying fuel and oxygen to the digestive process, too little is available for the brain and muscles. And when the brain does not get enough oxygen, the body falls asleep.

Combine starch, sugar, and water in a dark, warm environment and fermentation will invariably be the result. Fermentation produces two by-products: alcohol and gas. Alcohol in your system is harmful to you, invariably lowers performance abilities, and can prove deadly. No one wants to notice your gas.

To understand the principles of proper food combining, it is necessary to know something about the digestive process. The various chemical digestive functions occur in different parts of the digestive system and at different pH levels. In health, the pH of the mouth usually is slightly alkaline, about 7.4. The mouth, teeth, and tongue are primarily responsible for the mechanical digestion of the food, though some mechanical digestion also occurs in the stomach.

While the chewing process is occurring, the taste buds relay messages to the brain, which alerts the rest of the digestive system to get ready for action. A few substances can be absorbed directly into the bloodstream through the surface microcapillaries directly under the tongue. These include, but are not limited to, vitamin B-12, alcohol, and glucose.

Actual chemical digestion in the mouth is somewhat restricted and carried out in two ways. There is the secretion of saliva, which helps liquefy food, and in it is a small amount of salivary amylase, a starch-digesting enzyme. (Many ripe fruits and vegetables contain minute amounts of starch because the entire fruit does not ripen at the same time. The amylase production in the mouth is sufficient to break this starch down from its initial form as a complex carbohydrate to the simple carbohydrates required for uptake.) All starch digestion ceases in the presence of acids, however, because the ability of amylase to function is neutralized in the presence of acids. When foods mixed with salivary amylase reach the stomach, which is highly acidic, starch digestion comes to an abrupt halt. It will resume, but to a much lesser extent, when the starchy foods enter the small intestine.

> The mono meal is the rule in nature. Bears eat honey, and bears eat fish, but they never eat the two together. Squirrels eat berries, and squirrels eat nuts, but they never eat the two at the same time. Monkeys eat bananas, and monkeys eat seeds, but they never sit down and eat a complex meal. If we wish to stretch the limits of nature's guidelines, we must do so with extreme respect for the consequences.

The hydrochloric acid found in the stomach begins the digestion of proteins and fats. Large protein molecules are chemically broken down into smaller ones on their way to being fragmented by the liver into individual amino acids. In the same way that starch digestion cannot occur in the presence of acids, protein digestion cannot occur in the presence of an alkaline. The degree of alkalinity of the mouth and intestines and the degree of acidity of the stomach are affected by the nature of the foods consumed.

The stomach's acid can be 10 to 100 times stronger when protein foods are consumed than it is when carbohydrates are eaten. The pH of the mouth can also change to become several times more acidic or alkaline. One of the greatest challenges to digestion comes when foods that are predominantly starchy are consumed at the same time as foods that are concentrated with proteins. Neither the mouth's alkalinity nor the stomach's acidity can function at full strength, because both are being given mixed messages. The invariable result is poor or compromised digestion, with both proteins and starches being only partially digested, at best. Digestive distress is never supportive of athletic performance and should be considered worthy of avoiding.

Continuing to stress the digestive capacities beyond their maximum leads to a variety of digestive ailments far worse than just plain indigestion. The list of performance setbacks that can be caused by poor food combining is a literal A to Z of digestive ailments, including but certainly not limited to appendicitis, colitis, constipation, Crohn's disease, diarrhea, diverticulitis, diverticulosis, duodenal ulcer, gall stones, gastritis, GERD, heartburn, hepatitis, IBS, Ménétrier's disease, pancreatitis, peptic ulcer, polyps, proctitis, spastic colon syndrome, ulcerative colitis, and ZES.

> Can food ever taste good enough to make up for the indigestion and reduced performance ability it causes? Food always tastes better when you know that the consequences of eating it will support your health, performance, and life goals.

The stark truth of proper food combining contradicts the manner in which most of us have been taught to eat almost every meal of our lives. Virtually every traditional meal in our society combines a protein with a starch. Chicken and rice, steak and potatoes, pasta and cheese, cereal and milk, and bread and lunchmeat may be terrific when it comes to taste, but they are terrible when it comes to digestibility. The resulting digestive distress that will follow the consumption of these combinations is a foregone conclusion.

These meals do not digest well. They invariably require excessive quantities of time and effort by the entire digestive system. They always sit long and heavy in the stomach, and they do not yield up their full complement of nutrients. Simply look at how people feel after consuming a typical meal. Eight out of ten people have digestive troubles. Digestive problems keep doctors in business. The best-selling over-the-counter drugs, as well as the most commonly prescribed drugs, are for digestive disorders. More surgeries are performed for digestive disorders than for any other reason. Cancers of the digestive system are on a sharp upswing in frequency. Is it possible that so many people simply have bad stomachs? Or is it more likely that they have been trained to consistently and persistently do bad things to their stomachs?

Another common experience with the poor combination of starch and protein comes from eating mature legumes. Beans are an almost equal caloric combination of starch and protein. And what happens when people eat beans? They get foul gas, indigestion, and eventually, they suffer from poor fecal elimination. Nature has created many foods that are excellent for creatures with compatible digestive tracts but are poor choices for human beings. Legumes are a prime example. Mature beans are simply not an ideal food for humans, and they help prove the concept that eating starches and proteins together is never a good idea.

Starches combined with sugary foods will always spell digestive trouble as well. Pastry desserts fall into this category, as do sweet breakfast bars and sugary breakfast cereals. Look no farther than the local brewery to understand what happens to starches and sugars when they are mixed together. Breweries combine starch (barley) with sugar (malt), and then they wait for the fermentation to begin.

Proteins, on the other hand, do not ferment, but they do rot. The rotting process for proteins is referred to as "putrefaction." Imagine taking a piece of meat and putting it in a hot, humid, dark place for a couple of days. It rots, and it stinks. Because of a lack of fiber, animal proteins typically take two or three days to pass through the human digestive tract (often they can take a week and longer), a passage that is hot, humid, and dark. When the rotted protein finally hits the air, passed as fecal matter, the sheer stench of it tells the entire story all by itself.

> Amazingly, the expression, "Mine don't stink," is true for people who combine their foods properly.

There is a great deal more to be said about proper food combining and its implications to benefit the athlete. Improved digestion, enhanced nutrition, and an increased sense of energy are reason enough to embrace a new way of eating. Try it as an experiment for a month or two, and then you can judge the concept by your own results.

Basic Food Combining Guidelines:

1. If you eat starchy foods, eat them with raw vegetables, and in a separate meal from concentrated protein foods.
2. If you eat starchy foods, eat them in a separate meal from sweet foods, including sweet fruit.
3. If you eat starchy foods, do not eat them with vinegar or with highly acidic fruits.
4. Proteins combine best with raw vegetables and/or acid fruits. They do not combine well with starches, melons, or sweet fruits.
5. Fruits with a high-water content do not combine well with low-water content fruits.
6. Lettuce and celery combine well with everything.

> Good food combinations taste delicious, equally as good as the food you were brought up on. The difference is that they support you in going where you are trying to go. Go to health!

72

Chapter Fifteen

BANANAS AND ...

Bananas and Energy—Bananas are one of the world's finest foods for providing fuel for energy. They contain a unique blend of vitamins, minerals, and carbohydrates that foster a quick and efficient conversion to usable fuel. Whether a quick release of energy or a long-lasting supply of energy is needed, bananas supply the right fuel for the occasion. They contain two types of sugars: glucose and fructose. Because glucose is the most easily digestible sugar, it is released into the bloodstream rapidly for a quick burst of energy. Fructose is absorbed somewhat more slowly and provides a more lasting fuel release. Neither of these natural sugars causes the adrenaline surge associated with the consumption of sucrose (table sugar), and the fiber in the banana further moderates the uptake of the banana's sugars to make them ideal.

Because our bodies work to convert all food matter into simple carbohydrates (sugars) for use as fuel, the digestive processes themselves can require considerable fuel and energy and leave a person feeling tired. Some foods, such as many of the leafy vegetables, actually require more fuel to digest than the fuel they give back in return. And some people, especially those with chronic fatigue, simply do not have the ability to expend the energy required to deal with foods that are difficult to digest.

The carbohydrates in ripe bananas are already in their simplest form and can be digested with a minimum output of energy and fuel. Bananas are famous for their high levels of potassium, a mineral involved in proper muscle contraction. Insufficient potassium is one of the main causes of fatigue, muscle cramping, and dehydration, especially when it comes to physical performance.

Bananas also supply the dense and ready source of carbohydrates needed to replace the muscle glycogen (muscle sugar) used during exercise. It is wise to eat bananas, before, during, and after long bouts of activity, and immediately after shorter, more intense sessions. One meal a day of bananas is enough for most people, but many athletes, especially those eating four or more meals per day, find that two banana meals per day suits them just fine.

> Bananas aren't really all that special. Any relatively sweet fruit will do the job of nourishing an athlete. It is just that bananas are available year-round, tend to be inexpensive, give a reliable carbohydrate "hit," are easy to ripen, and can be found everywhere in the whole world. And they taste great!

Many people find that they fall into a pattern of eating. They have breakfast as a meal of high-water-content fruits, and dinner is a meal of acid fruit and high-volume vegetables. Lunch is their postworkout refueling, and it typically is a high-calorie meal of bananas, as many as they care for, or, as many as it takes to leave them satisfied until the next mealtime rolls around.

Bananas and Athletic Performance—Bananas are the perfect food for people with active lifestyles. They are self-contained, clean to eat, sweet, tasty, easy to eat in small or large quantities, satiating, available year-round, and inexpensive. Containing a near-perfect ratio of all nutrients, bananas provide almost all of an active person's food requirements. They are high in carbohydrates, typically containing two to four times as many carbohydrates per bite as most other fruits. A satiating meal of bananas provides enough fuel to remain active for hours, yielding up fuel for energy in a gradual manner.

During intense activities that last for more than 2 hours' duration (90 minutes at world-class levels of exertion), it is possible to drain the muscles of their fuel (glycogen) and begin to utilize the limited sugars in the bloodstream to feed the muscles. To prevent low blood sugar and the tired, sluggish feeling it brings, it is wise during exercise to consume a sports drink that's high in glucose. A banana or two blended into a quart of water will provide plenty of glucose to act as fuel for energy and will digest easily enough to prevent stomach problems. Each banana will supply sufficient fuel for approximately 5–15 (or more) minutes of continued exertion, depending upon the intensity level.

> Bicyclists who compete in some of the most rigorous competitions in the world have been famous for eating bananas for decades. Heck, their shirts are designed with "banana pockets" in the back.

To avoid fatigue after exercise, it is important to replenish muscle glycogen as soon as possible. Bananas are excellent for this as well. Although the fructose in bananas enters the bloodstream more slowly than the glucose, both are easily converted to muscle glycogen. The "glycemic index" tells how quickly the carbohydrates in foods are assimilated. Bananas are typically grouped with foods that have the highest glycemic index, or at the top of the middle group, and rate near the very top of the glycemic index of all fruits.

Bananas also have the best possible mix of vitamins, minerals, and enzymes for fueling activity. Their high potassium content (necessary for powerful muscular contractions) makes them the premier fruit for anyone who wishes to improve their nutrition and athletic performance. It is common for athletes to eat 10, 15, 20, and even a greater number of bananas a day.

The fact that bananas have an exceptionally low quantity of fat for their total calorie content contributes in two ways to making them ideal for sports performance. First, sports physiologists have proven that, in proportion to rises in levels of bloodstream fat, the ability of the blood to uptake, transport, and deliver oxygen to the cells falls. Getting oxygen to the cells is a primary concern for any active person. Second, and again, we can thank the sports physiologists for bringing this data to light and confirming it, the ability of the body to uptake, transport, and deliver fuel (glucose) to the cells is impaired in proportion to rises in bloodstream levels of fat. Essentially, as fat levels in the diet rise, athletic performance falls off.

> Bananas are to an athlete what prepackaged meals are to an astronaut … virtual survival. Yet athletes love their bananas as no astronaut has ever loved his prepackaged meals.

Bananas and Weight Loss—Bananas are the perfect food for someone who wants to lose weight. They are nutritious, delicious, and almost everyone likes them. Unlike celery and other "diet" foods, bananas are extremely satiating. Bananas are richer than most other fruits, providing the nutrient density needed to ensure proper nutrition while supplying the volume required to result in satiation. Fully ripened, they cause virtually no digestive problems, yet they take longer to pass through the stomach than fruits that are higher in water content. This combination of qualities yields a full, contented feeling for hours after eating a meal of bananas.

Most packaged foods are high in sodium, a mineral that causes water retention. Bananas are low in sodium but high in potassium. This ratio helps the body to bring back a healthy balance between these two minerals, and allows for the loss of excess water weight. Bananas provide such a healthy and well-balanced supply of vitamins and

> It is easy to picture a monkey eating a banana. Have you ever seen a fat monkey?

minerals that people have been known, in survival situations, to survive on a diet consisting solely of bananas for long periods of time, sometimes longer than a year.

Bananas contain several different carbohydrates that offer up their sugars at varying rates of speed. They satisfy quickly, and they give a satiation that is extremely long lasting. This makes it almost impossible to overeat on them. They also address a common cause of hunger, the lack of vitamins and minerals. Bananas contain a full complement of nutrients, and eating them is nutritionally sound. Many people find that by eating one meal of bananas per day that they can more easily control their weight than ever before.

BANANAS AND CANCER, HEART DISEASE, AND DIABETES

Cancer—All humans create, carry, and destroy cancer cells in their bodies every day. Typically, we destroy the cancer cells almost as quickly as we create them. It is only when production outpaces destruction that we get into trouble with cancer. In the same way that there are many causes of cancerous cells (foods, cooking options, radiation, airborne fumes and particulate matter, 'cides, chemicals, etc.), there are many lifestyle factors that help us eliminate cancer cells. Some of these influences include, but are certainly not limited to, sunlight, cardiovascular exercise, phytonutrients, free radicals (yes, free radicals are essential to our good health as well as being involved in losses of health), sufficient sleep, and fresh fruits and vegetables.

Bananas contain no known cancer-causing substances. In addition, many nutrient factors in bananas are considered to be anticancer agents. In preventing the onset of cancer or minimizing its spread, bananas are one of the world's best foods. Bananas are rich in nutrients known as antioxidants. These substances neutralize free radicals, which are proven cancer-causing agents. Current research suggests that there are also dozens, if not hundreds, of phytochemicals in bananas that play a role in cancer prevention.

Bananas are rich in soluble fiber. This type of fiber has anticancer properties both because it helps the colon keep itself clean, and because it encourages regularity by helping to keep the fecal mass water-rich.

Grains also have fiber, but it is the nonsoluble type, the kind that often irritates the digestive tract. Refined flours have their fiber removed in order to make these grain-based foods less irritating to the intestines, but then we are back to having the problem caused by eating foods that have limited quantities of fiber.

Eating several bananas per day, or more, will greatly reduce the risk of colon cancer and help reduce the risk of other cancers as well. For those already battling cancer, eating bananas every day helps reduce the spread and increases the chances of overcoming this dreaded condition. They are a low-fat fuel that makes for optimum oxygenation of all tissues, including cancerous ones. Low-fat diets have been proven optimum for cancer prevention and treatment protocols.

Heart Disease—Perhaps the biggest misconception that people have about heart disease is demonstrated by the fact that they are trying to cure it by eating certain foods. Heart disease is caused, and it is typically caused by the foods we choose. In order to free oneself of heart disease, it is not necessary to take the cure. All that is required is for us to stop causing (eating) the problem by not eating the problem foods. Therefore, a true understanding of heart disease allows us to eat any healthful foods that we desire. The trick to beating heart disease lies in the foods that we choose to eliminate from our diet, not in the foods that we eat.

> If a group of scientists with an unlimited budget got together to design the perfect nutritional supplement for preventing and reversing heart disease, they would predictably come up with the nutritional equivalent of the banana. And it would likely cost at least $20 per tablet.

Bananas are among the finest of all possible foods for sufferers of heart disease. They contain essentially no cholesterol, long known as one of the highest risk factors in heart disease. They also contain almost no fat, a feature that helps lower several other risk factors for heart disease. They do not cause one to become overweight, they aid in oxygen transport, and they have a positive effect on blood pressure. Perhaps more importantly, bananas are almost always eaten fresh and raw, features that lower the risk of heart disease by encouraging the blood to flow well.

It is estimated that although 65 percent of Americans die of heart disease, over 95 percent have some degree of this disabling condition. Bananas are a high-water-content food that is very low in sodium. These two features combine to keep the blood well hydrated, one of the most important factors in enabling efficient blood flow and controlling blood pressure. As the blood becomes dehydrated, it becomes thicker, causing blood pressure to rise dangerously. Cooked foods, even cooked bananas, elicit a flood of white blood cells into the bloodstream. The more solid material that is packed into the bloodstream, the higher blood pressure will tend to rise.

Bananas provide the simple carbohydrate fuel necessary for high-energy activities. Activity helps prevent heart disease in several ways. Exercising the heart muscle leads to a stronger heart, a lower resting heart rate, and contractions that are more effective. Exercise also increases the size and number of capillaries, making for more efficient blood flow. Lymphatic drainage is enhanced by muscular activity, resulting in improved protein and fat circulation, a factor that discourages blood thickening and helps to keep blood pressure under control.

Bananas are one of the best-known sources of the mineral potassium, necessary for proper contractions of the heart muscle. This, plus the serotonin in bananas, encourages strong and regular heartbeats and allows the heart to work properly even when it is under stress. Eating bananas on a daily basis is a good way to promote healthy heart tissue, to encourage good circulation, and to keep blood pressure down.

Diabetes—The trouble that most diabetics have (about 90 percent of all diabetics are Type II) isn't that they take in too much sugar; it is that they cannot effectively manage to get the sugar out of their blood. According to sports scientists, exercise physiologists,

> Even the American Diabetes Foundation recommends that diabetics eat all the fruit they desire. Why are doctors and raw food "authorities" still recommending that diabetics restrict their intake of fruit? Could it be that they want you to learn to live with diabetes, rather than putting it into your past?

and the medical professionals that have studied this issue, the biggest
obstacle to getting sugar out of the blood is the matter of having too
much fat circulating in the blood. By simply reducing the amount of
fat consumed to below 10 percent of calories consumed, almost all
Type II diabetics (these people can produce sufficient insulin, but the
insulin's function is somewhat reduced due to the effect of fats in the
bloodstream) will see instant improvements in their condition, if not
total erasure of all symptoms. The same has been shown to be true
for Type I diabetics (these people typically cannot produce sufficient
insulin to meet their requirements). They will all see improvements
and sometimes even erasure of their symptoms by switching to a
diet that is comprised of lower than 10 percent of calories from fat.
This information has been taught professionally since 1959.

Diabetics are often told to avoid bananas
entirely. Each person's case must be considered individually, of course, for some
people are truly allergic to bananas, but on
the whole, bananas are actually good for
the overwhelming majority of diabetics. The
fructose portion requires more time to get
into the bloodstream than the glucose. This,
coupled with the fact that a banana is
extremely low in fat, means that the sugar
can get into the bloodstream at a steady
pace, and, more importantly, that it can also
exit the bloodstream easily.

Guar gum and pectin are given to the diabetic in isolated form by medical doctors in order to help them control their blood sugar. Why is it that they simply do not suggest to their diabetic patients that they eat more fruit, the source of guar gum and pectin?

Bananas are high in soft, soluble fiber. When sugars are consumed with fiber, the sugar uptake is slowed down. The fiber in the
banana makes for a much more gradual uptake of sugar by the body
than when sucrose (table sugar) is consumed. This benefits diabetics,
as they can only handle sugar in relatively small, steady increments.
This gradual uptake means that diabetics are less likely to experience the damagingly high blood sugar levels that require surges
of insulin to be produced by the pancreas or for them to have to

take injections of insulin. They are also less likely to experience the extreme low blood sugar that also plagues diabetics who are not properly controlling their blood sugar level. Two of the specific "gums" in bananas that afford protection to the diabetic are guar gum and pectin. Both of these soluble fibers are known to be nutrients that slow down sugar uptake.

Bananas are rich in vitamins and minerals, making them a healthy choice for everyone. Eating even small amounts of bananas and a variety of other fruits each day is excellent for your health. And, because the results will be so rewarding, with practice, your banana consumption will increase, providing a nutritious and delicious food, even for diabetics.

> Life is meant to be sweet, even for a diabetic.

Chapter Sixteen
TIPS FOR ATHLETIC RECOVERY

1. Drink all the water you want before, during, and after strenuous activity. Becoming dehydrated will ALWAYS work against you.

2. Eat fruit after strenuous activity to bring your blood sugar back to normal levels and to provide sugar for conversion to muscle glycogen. Fruit will satiate like no other food can, and will help with your rehydration, as well.

3. Consume celery several times a week—or as often as you participate in strenuous activity—to provide the sodium you need. If celery doesn't seem appealing, be sure to consume other green, leafy vegetables.

4. Rest after meals to foster optimum digestion. Most people rest far too little. Resting after meals will help you to develop this worthwhile skill.

5. Remember that exercise does not provide energy, but that it requires energy. Sleep as much as you desire. Almost everyone allows themselves insufficient sleep. You will likely be shocked by how

> Eat like a champion every day, at every meal, and very soon, you will realize that it is not a hardship. In fact, feeling great is the reward, not the penalty. It is the people eating the same foods day in and day out, week in and week out, all year around, that are experiencing hardship. That is why they pick on you and your food, so that you won't pick on them.

much you will sleep if you give yourself the chance to sleep all you want.

6. During activities of long duration, drink homemade sports drinks of fresh whole fruit blended with water. For events of four or more hours in duration, add celery or celery juice to the mixture. Experiment with a variety of fruits until you find the one(s) that work best for you in various situations.

7. Monitor your water losses by using a scale to measure your weight before and after workouts. Replace lost water as soon as possible. This should be done by first drinking water and then by consuming juicy fruit.

8. Raw fruits and vegetables provide a nutrient ratio that most closely approximates our nutrient needs and encourages the most rapid recovery. Gradually increase the percentage of raw foods in your diet until you approach or reach 100 percent. The better you eat, the better you will play, whatever your activity choice may be.

9. Develop the habit of going to bed early to obtain a full night's sleep. There is a saying that the hours of sleep BEFORE midnight are the most valuable. It is more likely accurate that the more sleep you get before midnight, the better your chance of getting a full night's sleep by morning.

10. Keep meals simple for optimum digestion, absorption, assimilation, and elimination. Fruit meals need only one type of fruit per meal. No more than six ingredients are necessary for a great salad meal, including the dressing. Use a blender to blend one type of fat—avocado, nuts, or seeds—with one type of acid fruit—such as tomato, orange, or strawberry—for a delicious dressing. Or make fat-free dressings from a blend of vegetables and fruit, such as mango/tomato, berry/celery, or pineapple/pepper.

11. Vary the foods you consume throughout the year to ensure optimum nutrition. Eating with the seasons will

insure that you are getting the highest quality produce at the lowest cost. It will also give you more

> The mono meal is the ultimate ideal.

variety than if you attempt to eat the same foods all year around.

12. Strive for simplicity in your meals and variety in your diet.

Chapter Seventeen

SAMPLE MEALS FOR ATHLETES

When it comes right down to it, nutrition and athletic performance have a lot to do with eating the right foods, and eating
enough of them. Athletes tend to be very hungry come mealtime,
and they tend to eat more food, in total, than their sedentary counterparts. If an athlete doesn't take the time and make the effort to
learn to eat the *good* stuff, then s/he is likely to become very
tempted to eat the *other* stuff, foods that do not support optimum
athletic performance.

The beauty of eating properly is that there is more variety in a
seasonal diet of fruits and vegetables than there is in any other way
of eating. After all, a pizza tastes the same all year long. A hamburger
from a specific fast-food outlet tastes the same all year long, in every
part of the country. Canned beans, frozen orange juice, a box of
cereal, and every other prepared, packaged food tastes exactly the
same, all the time, wherever you go.

But even the same variety of fresh tomatoes tastes different during different times of the year, and from different parts
of the country. And there are dozens of varieties of tomatoes to
choose from.

Likewise, there are lots of varieties of melons, citrus, apples,
pears, grapes, mangoes, and other fruits to enjoy during the course
of their season, and each has a unique, distinctive flavor. Several
dozen types of salad greens, many kinds of cucumbers, and over a
dozen varieties of berries await the hungry consumer. Most large

grocery stores even carry six or so types of bananas. In our local store, I have seen Cavendish, Jamaican Red, Blue Java, Orinoco, Hawaiian, Mysore, and Apple bananas, to name just a few. A wonderful taste surprise awaits you with every bite of food you eat. The turn of each season brings new fruits and vegetables for consumption. Eating whole,

> When you decide to eat from the garden of earthly delights, you never really know what is going to be for dinner until you go out there and pick it. Happy gardening.

fresh, ripe, raw, organic fruits and vegetables, in season, offers an endless string of delicious and nutritious taste treats to delight the palate.

Breakfast—If you are at all thirsty, or believe you might become thirsty before you get back from your morning's activities, start the day with as much water as you desire. After your morning workout, eat a mono meal of one type of juicy fruit until you are satiated. Citrus, melon, pineapple, strawberry, papaya, mango, peach, or any other juicy fruit make excellent choices. Eat until you are satiated, until you are sure you have lost your appetite. You will know that you have eaten enough if the meal keeps you satiated until lunchtime. Developing the skill to eat enough breakfast may take some practice. If you get hungry between breakfast and lunch, either have another breakfast, or have an early lunch. Either way, let it be a learning experience, teaching you to eat sufficiently at breakfast time. It is likely that you will have to readjust your perceptions in terms of how much volume of food to eat in order to consume a meal that is satisfactorily satiating.

> What's for breakfast?
> A bowl of freshly diced mangoes and raspberries
> What's for lunch?
> Bananas, dates, and celery
> What's for dinner?
> Diced pineapple, tangerine slices, and a lettuce, tomato, red cabbage salad dressed with red pepper and kiwi, blended

Lunch—Lunch often follows another period of activity. Drink as much water as you want at least 10 minutes before your meal. Sweet fruits allow for the most calorie consumption with the fewest bites, and tend to be higher on the glycemic index. Bananas make the easiest and most predictably satiating meal, but any fruit will do the job. A meal of sweet or subacid fruits from the listing of common fruits (below) is also a good choice. Lettuce and/or celery with any of these fruits do a good job of increasing the mineral content of the meal and cutting the sweetness. Eat until you are fully satisfied. It is very common for athletes to make a meal of any one fruit and then follow that meal with as many bananas as is required to reach total satiation.

Dinner—If you are a truly active person, it is advisable to begin your evening meal with as much acid or subacid fruit as you want. Don't hold back. It might surprise you how much you want, but have all you desire. If you wish to limit your caloric intake, you may choose to skip the evening fruit. But be aware that skipping or skimping on the evening's fruit will likely leave you craving "something" at the end of the meal, and most likely, you will be driven to eat nuts or other concentrated fatty foods in quantities you didn't intend to. A large salad of lettuce, tomato, celery, and other vegetables, if desired, such as broccoli, cauliflower, asparagus, and red bell pepper should make up the main course. A dressing of an acid fruit blended with some vegetables is delicious. Feel free to experiment. As an option, a small quantity of avocado, nuts, or seeds may be added to the salad dressings on occasion.

Note: Athletes who need to consume over 4,000 calories a day may find that three meals per day are insufficient, and they may wish to add an extra meal. Bananas make the most effective and satiating extra meal. They supply approximately 90 calories per banana. It is common for athletes to eat from 10 to 20 bananas at one sitting, and sometimes more.

To determine the sufficiency of your meals, use the following statements as a general guideline.

- If you finish the meal and still want something sweet, you did not eat enough fruit at the start of the meal. In this instance, have more fresh fruit.

- If you finish the meal and still want something starchy, you did not eat enough fruit at the start of the meal. In this instance, have more fresh fruit.
- If you finish the meal and still want something heavy or rich, you did not eat enough fruit at the start of the meal. In this instance, have more fresh fruit.

> With practice, you will learn how much fruit to eat at each meal so that it will satiate you until the next meal. Eat until you are completely satiated and then practice, practice, practice. What fun!

- If you are craving refined sweets in between meals, you did not eat enough fresh fruit at the previous meal.

A LISTING OF SOME COMMON FRUITS BY CATEGORY

Melons—Canary, Cantaloupe, Casaba, Crenshaw, Galia, Honeydew, Persian, Santa Claus, Sharlyn, Watermelon

Acid Fruits—Blackberry, Carambola, Currant, Grapefruit, Gooseberry, Jostaberry, Kiwi, Kumquat, Lemon, Lime, Orange, Passion Fruit, Pineapple, Pomegranate, Pommelo, Raspberry, Strawberry, Tamarind, Tangerine

Subacid Fruits—Apple, Apricot, Blueberry, Cherry, Grape, Guava, Loquat, Mango, Mulberry, Nectarine, Papaya, Peach, Pear, Plum

Sweet Fruits—Banana, Breadfruit, Canistel, Cherimoya, Date, Fig, Jakfruit, Lychee, Mammea, Persimmon, Plantain, Rolinea, Sapodilla, Sugar Apple

Fatty Fruits—Akee, Avocado, Champedak, Durian, Olive

Vegetable Fruits—Cucumber, Eggplant, Okra, Pepper, Squash (winter and summer), Tomato

Chapter Eighteen

SPORTS DRINKS

In 1958, a salty-sweet beverage named Bengal Punch made its debut on the playing fields of the Louisiana State University campus. This is, most likely, the earliest reference to what eventually became known commercially as the "sports drink."

The purpose of a sports drink is to keep an athlete's supply of water, sugar, and electrolytes at an optimal level during long periods of activity. Typically, "long periods of activity" refers to sessions of activity having a minimum duration of longer than 1 hour, and commonly longer than 2 hours. There are also influencing factors to be considered, such as the intensity level of the exertion, sun, temperature, altitude, wind, and humidity. Since about 1990, sports drinks have gained worldwide attention and have received a tremendous amount of marketing. Unfortunately, the marketing of the product has superseded its ability to live up to the hype it is given.

Specialization in the field of sports drinks has resulted in two distinct types of drinks in addition to the general sports drink: the electrolyte replacement fluid and the hydration replacement fluid. Typically, the electrolyte replacement fluid is a salty drink that has few, if any, carbohydrates, and the hydration replacement fluid, though still mildly salty, is less so. As discussed in the chapter on mineral salts, electrolytes are important because they are what your cells

> A well-trained athlete, properly fueled, is able to go and go and go, and just keep on going. Truly the only thing that will stop such an athlete is the need for sleep.

use to maintain voltages across their cell membranes and to carry electrical impulses such as nerve impulses and muscle contractions across themselves and to other cells.

The major electrolytes found in your body are as follows (though in this book, as with most sports drinks, the focus with be only on sodium and potassium):

sodium (Na^+)

potassium (K^+)

chloride (Cl^-)

calcium (Ca^{2+})

magnesium (Mg^{2+})

bicarbonate (HCO_3^-)

phosphate (PO_4^{2-})

sulfate (SO_4^{2-})

Although sports scientists know that water quenches thirst best, marketers have discovered that athletes will drink more water if it is laced with salt. Even though everyone knows that when you add salt to water, the net result is one of dehydration, the marketers claim that because there is salt in the water, the athlete will drink more water, thus becoming better hydrated than if s/he solely drinks water. We know, due to the number of people who have died from drinking seawater, that this theory is seriously flawed, and that it is strictly to be viewed as nothing more than marketing jargon. We also know that if given a chance, the body will quickly adapt to a diet that includes no additional salt other than that which is found naturally in fruits and vegetables. It does so by reducing the quantity of sodium that is lost through perspiration to amounts that can be replaced through our food. This adaptation process whereby the

The all-time best, number one, undefeated champion hydration drink is—and always will be—WATER. Just plain old water cannot be beaten.

body regulates and reduces the amount of sodium lost through perspiration typically takes only about 3 weeks from start to finish.

Sports scientists have demonstrated that fit athletes use carbohydrates during sustained vigorous exercise at a rate of approximately 3 to 4 grams per minute. They have also concluded that the typical functional level of carbohydrates for an adult male athlete weighing 154 pounds is close to 400 grams of muscle glycogen. A female athlete weighing 132 pounds carries roughly 300 grams of fuel as muscle glycogen. This means that at full exertion, it is unlikely that an athlete is going to last 2 hours without reaching a point of almost complete exhaustion of fuel, an experience known as "hitting the wall." In order to continue exerting at maximum levels for longer periods of time, the athlete is obligated to refuel "on the go."

Scientists also teach that simple sugars are the best at satisfying the sense of hunger. They found that if the sports drink was sweet, athletes would drink less of it than if it was not sweet, so they used the same rationale as they did with salt (adding sugar to water means that even more water is needed in order to quench thirst). Therefore, they created a drink that contains (tasteless) complex sugars rather than a sweet-tasting drink in order to get the athletes to consume a greater quantity of their drink. Thus, they created a formula for the modern sports drink that has been duplicated around the world: salt water (that doesn't satisfy thirst) and laboratory-created polymer complex carbohydrates (that don't satisfy appetite), plus a few extra minerals such as potassium for electrolytes. Mix them together and voilà, you have a "sports drink" that will sell, and sell repeatedly, largely because it doesn't ever satisfy, so the consumer keeps drinking more of it. Sales, rather than customer satisfaction, is the key focus.

There are three types of sports drinks commonly in use today: isotonic, hypertonic, and hypotonic. Isotonic sports drinks contain proportions of water and other nutrients similar to those found in the human body. Hypertonic sports drinks contain a lesser proportion of water and a greater proportion of sugar than found in the human body. Hypotonic sports drinks contain a greater proportion of water and a lesser proportion of sugar than is commonly found in the human body.

> There is a sports drink that is even less complicated to make than bananas blended with lots of water. Blended watermelon. The pulp may be filtered out, if you wish, through a strainer, though it is not necessary. This drink works like a charm.

All of the chemistry, high-tech research, and fancy packaging can be bypassed to the ultimate benefit of the athlete. The simplest, healthiest, and most effective sports drinks are easy to make at home. Just blend a few bananas into a quart of water. This supplies water, sugar (glucose and fructose), and electrolytic minerals with enough vitamins and enzymes to properly metabolize them. The ratio of bananas to water can be regulated; custom-fit to meet the needs of any specific workout. An indoor strength workout may demand more sugar and less water. A hot weather endurance workout may require more water and electrolytes, but less sugar. To supply extra electrolytes without adding extra sugar, simply blend a stalk of celery into the mix. (Depending upon the nature of the activity, some athletes prefer to use celery juice rather than whole celery stalks.)

> The electrolyte content of one bite of a banana and one bite of celery exceeds the electrolyte content of most commercial electrolyte replacement drinks.

Another method of making a sports drink involves soaking a cup of dried fruit (raisins, figs, pineapples, or dates work well) overnight in a quart of water. The sugars and electrolytes in the fruit will mix into the water due to osmotic pressure. In the morning, pour the water into a container and you will have an excellent, instant sports drink. The richness of the drink can be controlled to meet individual requirements by simply changing the ratio of fruit to water. It is wise, when participating in activities that will last for many hours, to begin drinking a sports drink within 30 to 40 minutes of initiating the workout, and to continue drinking it until the activity is completed.

Chapter Nineteen

THE VEGETARIAN ATHLETE

Vegetarian, vegan, and raw food athletes are becoming more common in today's competitive sports world. They have broken into sports where people said it was impossible. Baseball, basketball, and football have always had the odd vegetarian player, but now, vegans and raw food athletes participate in these sports, too, at the highest professional level. Someday, they will be the norm, for they tend to outperform their meat-eating counterparts in a variety of ways. One of the most important ways is their reduced incidence of injury. In time, athletes always turn to that which works the best.

To be on the cutting edge of nutrition and performance demands that athletes supply themselves with the highest quality nutrients available. Without question, the highest quality nutrients are found in the greatest abundance in raw fruits and vegetables. In the sixties, a good pregame meal was thought to be steak and potatoes, with emphasis on the steak. Thirty years later, it was thought to be pasta, vegetables, and a bit of meat, but the lion's share of the meal was the pasta. The ideal pregame meal of the future will be the most nutritious and delicious of all, and will support performance like no other food can. It will consist primarily of fruit and plenty of green vegetables—and will be 100 percent raw. Cooked food will become passé for athletes—part of their history and nothing more. When athletes find a better way, they use it.

"I know I have to develop my abilities by training, but I also have to eat. Is it really possible for me to be my best, to improve my endurance, strength, and speed by eating nothing but fruits, vegetables, nuts, and seeds?" This is a common question when athletes express concern about the relationship of nutrition to their particular type of fitness. The answer is as unequivocal as it is simple: "Yes." Of course, training results depend upon training, too, and not only upon eating correctly.

Are you looking to become an athlete of the future, setting the example with your exemplary eating habits, or are you going to wait until the leaders pass you by, and then try to catch up?

The question, however, is asked in a completely backward form. The more logical question would be, "Is it possible to reach my full athletic potential on a diet to which my body is not biologically adapted? What if I eat a diet that includes very little whole, fresh, ripe, raw, organic fruits and vegetables? Can I actually perform at the top of my game and still smoke cigarettes, drink alcohol, eat the flesh, milk, and eggs of animals, consume grains and other complex carbohydrates, rely upon stimulants, irritants, supplements, and condiments, and while I am at it, have all the candy, recreational drugs, chocolate, and whatever else I desire?"

Again, the answer is certain and simple: "No." From a physiological perspective, it's like asking if it's possible to reach one's full athletic potential if one trains only infrequently, on a random basis. In order to thrive athletically, every person requires sufficient sleep; a diet predominated by, if not composed of, 100 percent raw fruits and vegetables; and must fully and regularly participate in a system of intelligently designed training procedures and practices.

If athletes trained in the way that most nonathletes do, they would be in the same out-of-shape physical condition as most other people. And if athletes ate like most nonathletes, they would come to expect the same food-related health problems as most other people. Let's be perfectly honest here. The majority of conservative medical doctors openly express their view that 90 percent of all illness is nutritionally related. The more open-minded and forward-thinking doctors, the ones considered "radicals" in their field, and the ones getting the best results, say that 98–99 percent of all illnesses could be avoided if we simply changed the way we eat. And they all stress the importance of whole, fresh, ripe, raw, organic fruits and vegetables.

It is interesting to note that, for the most part, athletes do not experience any major health advantages over most Americans, other than their fitness itself. They die of heart disease at about the same rate as nonathletes. The occurrence of diabetes is just as common for athletes as for anyone else. The cancer rate for athletes is higher than the mainstream, and they tend to develop that cancer at a younger age. Of course, their "wear and tear" type injury rate is much greater than that of nonathletes. Overall, being an athlete infers no specific health advantages, at least not the way athletes are currently taking care of themselves.

> In order to train like a champion, one must eat like a champion.

Doesn't it seem strange that athletes should be expected to eat the same way as everyone else? We certainly do not put the same fuel in a high-performance racing car as we put in the family car. We don't feed a thoroughbred racehorse the same food as we do a backyard pony. Why should we recommend the standard American diet (SAD) to the athlete? In fact, it is the very fact that athletes eat so much more food than most people that they need to make the choice to eat high-quality food. The toxins, pesticides, mutagens, carcinogens, antinutrients, and empty calories all take their toll on us based on their volume to which we are exposed. Therefore, because athletes eat more food than everyone else, it is they who are at the greatest risk of running into health problems caused by toxins in their

> Look around you. Vegans are popping up everywhere. "Show me the money," as the saying goes. If one were to consider all factors, there is only one inescapable conclusion: vegan and raw-vegan athletes so dominate all fields of athletic endeavor that to try to reach the top of any competitive sport without becoming a raw vegan would be sheer madness. It is time to raise the bar on your commitment to fitness.

food. Sure, being fit offers a bit of protection against disease, especially when compared to those who are unfit. But based on the disease rates, and especially the cancer rates, it would be unwise to suggest that athletes do not need to pay attention to their diets.

Few if any sports require only one aspect of fitness. Most demand complex combinations of speed, strength, endurance, agility, balance, coordination, flexibility, awareness, and many other qualities. Every aspect of fitness is directly affected by the quality of the diet, or lack thereof, and improves as the diet becomes more closely aligned with the foods to which we are biologically adapted. How long do you think it will be before the low-fat, raw, vegan athlete becomes the rule, rather than the exception? How long will it take *you* to join the leaders?

Athlete	Sport, Game, or Event
Henry Aaron	Baseball
Ridgely Abele	Karate
B. J. Armstrong	U.S. basketball star
Al Beckles	Bodybuilder
Surya Bonaly	Olympic figure skating champion
Les Brown	Veteran runner
Peter Burwash	Tennis
Andreas Cahling	Bodybuilding champion
Chris Campbell	1980 World Champion wrestler
Austin Carr	Cleveland Cavaliers pro basketball team
Rudy Carti	World record for 151,000 abdominal crunches in 48 hours
Nicky Cole	First woman to walk to the North Pole
Joanna Conway	Ice skater
Sylvia Cranston	Triathlete

Athlete	Sport, Game, or Event
Sally Eastall	Marathon runner—UK No. 2, vegan
Di Edwards	Runner, Olympic semifinalist
Cory Everson	Bodybuilder, Ms. Olympia 6 times
Katie Fitzgibbon	Marathon runner
Clare Francis	Sailor
Louis Freitas	Bodybuilder
Goose Gossage	San Diego Padres
Carol Gould	Marathon runner
Ronnie Grandison	NBA basketball
Estelle Gray & Cheryl Marek	Cross-country tandem cycling
Sammy Green	Runner
Dick Gregory	Trained at the University of Illinois, ran 3,000 miles across the USA on a fruitarian diet
Ruth Heidrich	3-time Ironman finisher, marathoner, age-group record holder, Pres. Vegetarian Society of Honolulu
Sally Hibberd	British women's mountain bike champion
Roy Hilligan	Bodybuilding
Keith Holmes	World Champion middleweight boxer
Sharon Hounsell	Miss Wales Bodybuilding Champion
Desmond Howard	Jacksonville Jaguars
Roger Hughes	Welsh National Ski Champion
Peter Hussing	European super heavyweight boxing champion
David Johnson	BAA coach
Kathy Johnson	Olympic gymnast
Alan Jones	British ski jumper
Billie-Jean King	Tennis champion
"Killer" Kowalski	Pro wrestling

Continued

Athlete	Sport, Game, or Event
Donnie LaLonde	Former light heavyweight champion of the world. Lost title to Sugar Ray Leonard
Tony LaRussa	Manager of St. Louis Cardinals—U.S. team
Silken Laumann	Olympic rower
Debbie Lawrence	World record holder, women's 5K race walk
Judy Leden	British, European & World Hang Gliding Champion
Marv Levey	Buffalo Bills coach
Carl Lewis	Olympic long jump and sprint
Jack Maitland	Triathlete and fell-runner
Ingra Manecki	World Champion discus thrower
Bill Manetti	Power-lifting champion
Leslie Marx	Fencer;1996 women's épée national champion
Ben Matthews	U.S. Master's Marathon Champion
Kirsty McDermott	Runner
Lindford McFarquar	Bodybuilder
Robert Millar	Cyclist
Dan Millman	Gymnast and trampolinist
Katherine Monbiot	World Champion arm wrestler and nutritionist
Monika Montsho	Weight lifter, 2× runner-up GB championships, 60kg; NW woman weight lifter of the year, 1991
Edwin Moses	Olympic hurdler
Jutta Müller	Multiple windsurfing World Cup Champion
Julie Ann Niewiek	Basketball commentator
Paavo Nurmi	Olympic distance running
Robert Parish	Basketball
Jamie Parsley	Cycling
Walter Payton	American football

Athlete	Sport, Game, or Event
Bill Pearl	Bodybuilder, Mr. America
Anthony Peeler	NBA Grizzlies basketball player
Bill Pickering	British Channel swimmer
Peace Pilgrim	Vowed to walk 'til humankind found peace; not to eat unless offered food
Dennis Rodman	Basketball for Bulls
Murry Rose	Olympic Gold medalist, swimming
Dave Scott	6-time Hawaii Ironman
Debbie Spaeth-Herring	Georgia State power-lifter
Jonathan Speelman	Chess
Lucy Stephens	Triathlete—vegan
Art Still	Buffalo Bills and Kansas City Chiefs MVP defensive end, Kansas City Chiefs Hall of Fame
Robert Sweetgall	Utlra-distance walker
Jacques Vaughn	All-American point guard, #1-ranked University of Kansas
Kirsty Wade	Runner
Bill Walton	Basketball player
Johnnie Weissmuller	Olympic Gold medalist, swimming
Jane Wetzel	U.S. National Marathon Champion
Charlene Wong-Williams	Olympic Champion figure skater

All anthropoid primates are herbivores/ frugivores. Humans are classified as anthropoid primates and must be considered herbivores/frugivores from the standpoint of comparative anatomy. Animals that are anatomically and physiologically similar to one another require similar foods in order to thrive. Consider this comparative anatomy listing:

> Do you ever even stop to wonder why vegan and raw-vegan athletes are leading the way in virtually all sports disciplines?

Anthropoid Ape	Carnivore	Human
Walks upright	No	Yes
Two hands	No	Yes
Two feet	No	Yes
Forward vision	No	Yes
Millions of pores	No	Yes
Smooth tongue	No	Yes
Well-developed incisors	No	Yes
5*1*4*1*5 dental formula	No	Yes
Blunt molar teeth	No	Yes
Produces salivary amylase	No	Yes
Mammary gland on chest	No	Yes
Only two mammary glands	No	Yes
Disc-shaped placenta	No	Yes
Lacking claws	No	Yes
Flat nails	No	Yes
Lacking a tail	No	Yes
Long intestines, 12× body length	No	Yes
Stomach with duodenum	No	Yes
Relatively weak stomach acid	No	Yes
Convoluted colon	No	Yes

Anthropoid Ape	Carnivore	Human
Susceptible to cholesterol buildup	No	Yes
Sweats through the skin	No	Yes
Cools the body via perspiration	No	Yes
Low uric acid production	No	Yes
Low capacity for processing uric acid	No	Yes
Alkaline saliva	No	Yes
Alkaline blood	No	Yes
Alkaline urine	No	Yes
Urine has weak odor	No	Yes
Vertical and horizontal jaw movement	No	Yes
Pouchlike cheeks	No	Yes
Lips capable of manipulating food	No	Yes
Flattened facial structure	No	Yes
Drinks via suction	No	Yes

How is it possible for anyone to intelligently argue against the facts? How can an athlete read the above list and still enjoy cooked food, meat, bread, or any other substance that puts his/her athletic performance into a downspin and jeopardizes his/her entire career?

THOUGHTS IN CONCLUSION

The motto that "more is better" usually doesn't work. Certainly, it doesn't apply to human nutrition. Simply put, human beings need only enough nutrients for their bodies to function at optimal levels. Serious consideration must be given to the possibility that "more is worse," and that athletes and nonathletes alike should exhibit caution when considering "nutritional supplements" of any kind. Nutritional supplements could just as easily be referred to as "nutritional detriments." Would that change your feelings towards them?

Improved hygiene has raised the standard of living for many people, but the novel idea of "better living through chemistry" has turned out to be a myth. It's time to realize that very often, it is what we take *out* of our diet that counts more than what we add *in* to it. Without question, there are hundreds and even thousands of items in a typical athlete's diet that exert a detrimental influence upon athletic performance. It is incumbent upon every athlete to be aware, and take into consideration, that cooked food has lost almost all of its nutritional value before taking another bite. Additionally, cooked food has accumulated a wide array of health-destroying qualities through the application of heat, including many antinutrients, mutagens, and carcinogens. This puts even the most "healthy" of cooked foods into the same negative, not-to-be-consumed category, along with refined and processed foods. These primarily supply empty calories, empty promises, and negative nutrition.

The degree to which an athlete "cleans up" his or her diet has a direct correlation on the degree to which the athlete experiences improvement in every phase and aspect of physical performance. Although changes in diet may seem like enormous steps at first, the reality is that a gradual and

> Nutrition has never been easier or simpler: eat all the fresh fruits you care for, and all the raw vegetables you desire.

steady approach becomes easy and is speedy and effective over time. Changes of 2 percent a week become 100 percent in just 1 year. The easiest, shortest, and most successful transition, however, is always the most direct one.

It is helpful to note that once it is established, most people love their food regimen regardless of its content. This is true around the world, regardless of your diet, no matter how many times you change it. You inevitably come to love whatever dietary program you are currently following. This is a basic human characteristic and belies our upbeat nature. This phenomenon is similar to the way most people become truly enamored with their training routines, often looking forward to and enjoying intensities of activity that were once totally out of reach before they became adapted to them. People love to grow, to stretch, to learn. A dietary regimen that fulfils all nutritional needs, tastes great, is incredibly satiating, requires practically no preparation or clean-up time, results in no indigestion, no dirty dishes, no negative environmental impact, and perfectly supports athletic performance may not be every

> Aren't you now really just itching to find out for yourself whether a diet of whole, fresh, ripe, raw, organic fruits and vegetables is the best for your nutrition and athletic performance?

athlete's dream. But if all the diet did was to facilitate the athlete's achievement and performance goals better than any other diet, it would be worth a try to most athletes. Generally, athletes who try **The 80/10/10® Diet** absolutely love it, and they report noteworthy, objective, measurable, positive changes to their performance abilities in less than a month.

CHARTS

The following charts offer a comparison of nutrients for a variety of foods. As you will see, fruits and vegetables provide superior nutrition in a wide variety of categories.

Sweet Fruits, serving size 100 grams				
	Apple	**Banana**	**Blackberry**	**Blueberry**
Water, g	85.56	74.91	88.15	84.21
Calories	52	89	43	57
Carbohydrate*, g	13.81	22.84	9.61	14.49
Protein, g	0.26	1.09	1.39	0.74
Fat, g	0.17	0.33	0.49	0.33
Fiber, g	2.4	2.6	5.3	2.4
Cholesterol, mg	-	-	-	-
Calcium, mg	6	5	29	6
Iron, mg	0.12	0.26	0.62	0.28
Phosphorous, mg	11	22	22	12
Magnesium, mg	5	27	20	6
Sodium, mg	1	1	1	1
Potassium, mg	107	358	162	77
Niacin, mg	0.091	0.665	0.646	0.418
Riboflavin, mg	0.026	0.073	0.026	0.041
Vitamin A, IU	54	64	214	54
Vitamin C, mg	4.6	8.7	21	9.7
Vitamin B-6, mg	0.041	0.367	0.03	0.052

Sweet Fruits, serving size 100 grams				
	Cantaloupe	**Cherry, Sweet**	**Dates, Medjool**	**Fig**
Water, g	90.15	82.25	21.32	79.11
Calories	34	63	277	74
Carbohydrate*, g	8.16	16.01	74.97	19.18
Protein, g	0.84	1.06	1.81	0.75
Fat, g	0.19	0.2	0.15	0.3
Fiber, g	0.9	2.1	6.7	2.9
Cholesterol, mg	-	-	-	-
Calcium, mg	9	13	64	35
Iron, mg	0.21	0.36	0.9	0.37
Phosphorous, mg	15	21	62	14
Magnesium, mg	12	11	54	17
Sodium, mg	16	-	1	1
Potassium, mg	267	222	696	232
Niacin, mg	0.734	0.154	1.61	0.4
Riboflavin, mg	0.019	0.033	0.06	0.05
Vitamin A, IU	3382	64	149	142
Vitamin C, mg	36.7	7	-	2
Vitamin B-6, mg	0.072	0.049	0.249	0.113

Sweet Fruits, serving size 100 grams				
	Grapefruit, White	Grapes	Mango	Nectarine
Water, g	90.48	80.54	81.71	87.59
Calories	33	69	65	44
Carbohydrate*, g	8.41	18.1	17	10.55
Protein, g	0.69	0.72	0.51	1.06
Fat, g	0.1	0.16	0.27	0.32
Fiber, g	1.1	0.9	1.8	1.7
Cholesterol, mg	-	-	-	-
Calcium, mg	12	10	10	6
Iron, mg	0.06	0.36	0.13	0.28
Phosphorous, mg	8	20	11	26
Magnesium, mg	9	7	9	9
Sodium, mg	-	2	2	-
Potassium, mg	148	191	156	201
Niacin, mg	0.269	0.188	0.584	1.125
Riboflavin, mg	0.02	0.07	0.057	0.027
Vitamin A, IU	33	66	765	332
Vitamin C, mg	33.3	10.8	27.7	5.4
Vitamin B-6, mg	0.043	0.086	0.134	0.025

Sweet Fruits, serving size 100 grams			
	Orange, Valencia	Papaya	Peach	Persimmon
Water, g	87.59	88.83	88.87	80.32
Calories	44	39	39	70
Carbohydrate*, g	10.55	9.81	9.54	18.59
Protein, g	1.06	0.61	0.91	0.58
Fat, g	0.32	0.14	0.25	0.19
Fiber, g	1.7	1.8	1.5	3.6
Cholesterol, mg	-	-	-	-
Calcium, mg	6	24	6	8
Iron, mg	0.28	0.1	0.25	0.15
Phosphorous, mg	26	5	20	17
Magnesium, mg	9	10	9	9
Sodium, mg	-	3	-	1
Potassium, mg	201	257	190	161
Niacin, mg	1.125	0.338	0.806	0.1
Riboflavin, mg	0.027	0.032	0.031	0.02
Vitamin A, IU	332	1094	326	1627
Vitamin C, mg	5.4	61.8	6.6	7.5
Vitamin B-6, mg	0.025	0.019	0.025	0.1

Sweet Fruits, serving size 100 grams				
	Pineapple	Raspberry	Strawberry	Watermelon
Water, g	86	85.75	90.95	91.45
Calories	50	52	32	30
Carbohydrate*, g	13.12	11.94	7.68	7.55
Protein, g	0.54	1.2	0.67	0.61
Fat, g	0.12	0.65	0.3	0.15
Fiber, g	1.4	6.5	2	0.4
Cholesterol, mg	-	-	-	-
Calcium, mg	13	25	16	7
Iron, mg	0.29	0.69	0.41	0.24
Phosphorous, mg	8	29	24	11
Magnesium, mg	12	22	13	10
Sodium, mg	1	1	1	1
Potassium, mg	109	151	153	112
Niacin, mg	0.5	0.598	0.386	0.178
Riboflavin, mg	0.032	0.038	0.022	0.021
Vitamin A, IU	58	33	12	569
Vitamin C, mg	47.8	26.2	58.8	8.1
Vitamin B-6, mg	0.112	0.055	0.047	0.045

Vegetables, serving size 100 grams			
	Arugula/ Rocket	Broccoli	Cabbage, Green	Cabbage, Red
Water, g	91.71	89.3	92.18	90.39
Calories	25	34	25	31
Carbohydrate*, g	3.65	6.64	5.8	7.37
Protein, g	2.58	2.82	1.28	1.43
Fat, g	0.66	0.37	0.1	0.16
Fiber, g	1.6	2.6	2.5	2.1
Cholesterol, mg	-	-	-	-
Calcium, mg	160	47	40	45
Iron, mg	1.46	0.73	0.47	0.8
Phosphorous, mg	52	66	26	30
Magnesium, mg	47	21	12	16
Sodium, mg	27	33	18	27
Potassium, mg	369	316	170	243
Niacin, mg	0.305	0.639	0.234	0.418
Riboflavin, mg	0.086	0.117	0.04	0.069
Vitamin A, IU	2373	623	98	-
Vitamin C, mg	15	89.2	36.6	57
Vitamin B-6, mg	0.073	0.175	0.124	0.209

Vegetables, serving size 100 grams				
	Carrots	**Cauliflower**	**Celery**	**Collards**
Water, g	88.29	91.91	95.43	90.55
Calories	41	25	16	30
Carbohydrate*, g	9.58	5.3	2.97	5.69
Protein, g	0.93	1.98	0.69	2.45
Fat, g	0.24	0.1	0.17	0.42
Fiber, g	2.8	2.5	1.6	3.6
Cholesterol, mg	-	-	-	-
Calcium, mg	33	22	40	145
Iron, mg	0.3	0.44	0.2	0.19
Phosphorous, mg	35	44	24	10
Magnesium, mg	12	15	11	9
Sodium, mg	69	30	80	20
Potassium, mg	320	303	260	169
Niacin, mg	0.983	30	0.32	0.742
Riboflavin, mg	0.058	0.063	0.057	0.13
Vitamin A, IU	16706	13	449	6668
Vitamin C, mg	33	46.4	3.1	35.3
Vitamin B-6, mg	0.138	0.222	0.074	0.165

Vegetables, serving size 100 grams				
	Kale	**Lettuce, Romaine**	**Spinach**	**Tomato**
Water, g	84.46	94.61	91.4	94.5
Calories	50	17	23	18
Carbohydrate*, g	10.01	3.29	3.63	3.92
Protein, g	3.3	1.23	2.86	0.88
Fat, g	0.7	0.3	0.39	0.2
Fiber, g	2	2.1	2.2	1.2
Cholesterol, mg	-	-	-	-
Calcium, mg	135	33	99	10
Iron, mg	1.7	0.97	2.71	0.27
Phosphorous, mg	56	30	49	24
Magnesium, mg	34	14	79	11
Sodium, mg	43	8	79	5
Potassium, mg	447	247	558	237
Niacin, mg	1	0.313	0.724	0.594
Riboflavin, mg	0.13	0.067	0.189	0.019
Vitamin A, IU	15376	5807	9377	833
Vitamin C, mg	120	24	28.1	12.7
Vitamin B-6, mg	0.271	0.074	0.195	0.08

Fatty Fruits, Nuts, Seeds, Butters and Oils, serving size 100 grams				
	Almonds, Whole	Almond Butter	Avocado, CA	Avocado, FL
Water, g	4.7	1	72.33	78.81
Calories	21.67	633	167	120
Carbohydrate*, g	21.67	21.22	8.64	7.82
Protein, g	21.22	15.08	1.96	2.23
Fat, g	49.42	59.1	15.41	10.06
Fiber, g	12.2	3.7	6.8	5.6
Cholesterol, mg	-	-	-	-
Calcium, mg	264	270	13	10
Iron, mg	3.72	3.7	0.61	0.17
Phosphorous, mg	484	523	54	40
Magnesium, mg	268	303	29	24
Sodium, mg	1	11	8	2
Potassium, mg	705	758	507	351
Niacin, mg	3.385	2.875	1.463	0.672
Riboflavin, mg	1.014	0.611	0.143	0.053
Vitamin A, IU	1	-	147	140
Vitamin C, mg	-	0.7	8.8	17.4
Vitamin B-6, mg	0.143	0.076	0.287	0.078

Fatty Fruits, Nuts, Seeds, Butters and Oils, serving size 100 grams			
	Brazil Nuts	Cashews	Coconut Meat	Coconut Water
Water, g	3.48	5.2	46.99	94.99
Calories	656	553	354	19
Carbohydrate*, g	12.27	30.19	15.23	3.71
Protein, g	14.32	18.22	3.33	0.72
Fat, g	66.43	43.85	33.49	0.2
Fiber, g	7.5	3.3	9	1.1
Cholesterol, mg	-	-	-	-
Calcium, mg	160	37	14	24
Iron, mg	2.43	6.68	2.43	0.29
Phosphorous, mg	725	593	113	20
Magnesium, mg	376	292	32	25
Sodium, mg	3	12	20	105
Potassium, mg	659	660	356	250
Niacin, mg	0.295	1.062	0.54	0.08
Riboflavin, mg	0.035	1.062	0.02	0.057
Vitamin A, IU	-	-	-	-
Vitamin C, mg	0.7	0.5	3.3	2.4
Vitamin B-6, mg	0.101	0.417	0.054	0.032

Fatty Fruits, Nuts, Seeds, Butters and Oils, serving size 100 grams			
	Flaxseed	Hazelnuts	Macadamia	Oil, Coconut
Water, g	6.96	5.31	1.36	-
Calories	534	628	718	862
Carbohydrate*, g	28.88	16.7	1.14	-
Protein, g	18.29	14.95	7.91	-
Fat, g	42.16	60.75	75.77	100
Fiber, g	27.3	9.7	8.6	-
Cholesterol, mg	-	-	-	-
Calcium, mg	255	114	85	-
Iron, mg	5.73	4.7	3.69	0.04
Phosphorous, mg	642	290	188	-
Magnesium, mg	392	163	130	-
Sodium, mg	30	-	5	-
Potassium, mg	813	680	368	-
Niacin, mg	3.08	1.8	2.473	-
Riboflavin, mg	0.161	0.113	0.162	-
Vitamin A, IU	-	20	-	-
Vitamin C, mg	0.6	6.3	1.2	-
Vitamin B-6, mg	0.473	0.563	0.275	-

Fatty Fruits, Nuts, Seeds, Butters and Oils, serving size 100 grams				
	Oil, Olive	Olive, Canned	Pecan	Pine Nuts
Water, g	-	79.99	3.52	2.28
Calories	884	115	691	673
Carbohydrate*, g	-	6.62	13.86	13.08
Protein, g	-	0.84	9.17	13.69
Fat, g	100	10.68	9.17	68.37
Fiber, g	-	3.2	9.6	3.7
Cholesterol, mg	-	-	-	-
Calcium, mg	1	88	70	16
Iron, mg	0.56	3.3	2.53	5.53
Phosphorous, mg	-	3	277	575
Magnesium, mg	-	4	121	251
Sodium, mg	2	872	0	2
Potassium, mg	1	8	410	597
Niacin, mg	-	0.037	1.167	4.387
Riboflavin, mg	-	-	0.13	0.227
Vitamin A, IU	-	403	56	29
Vitamin C, mg	-	0.9	1.1	0.8
Vitamin B-6, mg	-	0.009	0.21	0.094

Fatty Fruits, Nuts, Seeds, Butters and Oils, serving size 100 grams				
	Pistachio	Pumpkin Seed	Tahini	Walnuts
Water, g	3.97	6.92	3	4.07
Calories	557	541	570	654
Carbohydrate*, g	27.97	17.81	26.19	13.71
Protein, g	20.61	24.54	17.81	15.23
Fat, g	44.44	45.85	48	65.21
Fiber, g	10.3	3.9	9.3	6.7
Cholesterol, mg	-	-	-	-
Calcium, mg	107	43	420	98
Iron, mg	4.15	14.97	2.51	2.91
Phosphorous, mg	490	1174	752	346
Magnesium, mg	121	535	96	158
Sodium, mg	1	18	74	2
Potassium, mg	1025	807	414	441
Niacin, mg	1.3	1.745	5.925	1.125
Riboflavin, mg	0.16	0.32	0.51	0.15
Vitamin A, IU	553	380	67	20
Vitamin C, mg	5	1.9	-	1.3
Vitamin B-6, mg	1.7	0.224	0.149	0.537

Animal Foods, serving size 100 grams				
	Beef, Top Sirloin	Beef, Ground	Butter, Salted	Cheese, Cheddar
Water, g	60.33	55.78	15.87	36.75
Calories	212	270	717	403
Carbohydrate*, g	-	-	0.06	1.28
Protein, g	29.33	25.56	0.85	24.9
Fat, g	9.67	17.86	81.11	33.14
Fiber, g	-	-	-	-
Cholesterol, mg	73	88	215	105
Calcium, mg	22	41	24	721
Iron, mg	1.89	2.48	0.02	0.68
Phosphorous, mg	229	202	24	512
Magnesium, mg	25	20	2	28
Sodium, mg	61	96	576	621
Potassium, mg	368	328	24	98
Niacin, mg	7.807	4.859	0.042	0.08
Riboflavin, mg	0.141	0.186	0.034	0.375
Vitamin A, IU	-	-	2499	0.375
Vitamin C, mg	-	-	-	-
Vitamin B-6, mg	0.614	0.429	0.003	0.074

Animal Foods, serving size 100 grams				
	Chicken, Breast	Chicken, Drumstick	Egg, Whole	Ham, Sliced
Water, g	62.44	66.74	75.84	67.27
Calories	197	172	143	163
Carbohydrate*, g	-	-	0.77	3.83
Protein, g	29.8	28.29	12.58	16.6
Fat, g	7.78	5.66	9.94	8.6
Fiber, g	-	-	-	1.3
Cholesterol, mg	84	93	423	57
Calcium, mg	14	12	53	24
Iron, mg	1.07	1.3	1.83	1.02
Phosphorous, mg	214	184	191	153
Magnesium, mg	27	24	12	22
Sodium, mg	71	95	140	1304
Potassium, mg	245	246	134	287
Niacin, mg	12.7	6.075	0.07	2.904
Riboflavin, mg	0.119	0.233	0.478	0.178
Vitamin A, IU	93	60	487	-
Vitamin C, mg	-	-	-	4
Vitamin B-6, mg	0.56	0.39	0.143	0.329

Animal Foods, serving size 100 grams				
	Milk. 2% Milkfat	Turkey, Breast	Salmon	Shrimp
Water, g	89.33	74.04	72	77.28
Calories	50	104	117	99
Carbohydrate*, g	4.68	4.21	-	-
Protein, g	3.3	17.07	18.28	20.91
Fat, g	1.97	1.66	4.32	1.08
Fiber, g	-	0.05	-	-
Cholesterol, mg	8	43	23	195
Calcium, mg	117	8	11	39
Iron, mg	0.03	1.44	0.85	3.09
Phosphorous, mg	94	162	164	137
Magnesium, mg	11	21	18	34
Sodium, mg	41	1015	784	224
Potassium, mg	150	302	175	182
Niacin, mg	0.092	0.11	4.72	2.59
Riboflavin, mg	0.185	0.32	0.101	0.032
Vitamin A, IU	189	33	87	225
Vitamin C, mg	0.2	5.7	-	2.2
Vitamin B-6, mg	0.038	0.128	0.278	0.127

Starchy Vegetables, Grains and Breads, serving size 100 grams			
	Amaranth	Barley, Pearled	Buckwheat	Bread (WW)
Water, g	9.84	68.8	9.75	32.7
Calories	374	123	343	278
Carbohydrate*, g	66.17	28.22	71.5	51.4
Protein, g	14.45	2.26	13.25	8.4
Fat, g	6.51	0.44	3.4	5.4
Fiber, g	9.3	3.8	10	6
Cholesterol, mg	-	-	-	-
Calcium, mg	153	11	18	33
Iron, mg	7.59	1.33	2.2	3.1
Phosphorous, mg	455	54	347	187
Magnesium, mg	266	22	231	81
Sodium, mg	21	3	1	346
Potassium, mg	366	93	460	314
Niacin, mg	1.286	2.063	7.02	3.985
Riboflavin, mg	0.208	0.062	0.425	0.227
Vitamin A, IU	-	7	-	3
Vitamin C, mg	4.2	-	-	-
Vitamin B-6, mg	0.223	0.115	0.21	0.199

Starchy Vegetables, Grains and Breads, serving size 100 grams				
	Rice, Brown	Rice, White	Spaghetti, Enriched	Sweet Potato
Water, g	72.96	68.61	62.13	75.78
Calories	112	130	158	90
Carbohydrate*, g	23.51	28.59	30.86	20.71
Protein, g	2.32	2.38	5.8	2.01
Fat, g	0.83	0.21	0.93	0.15
Fiber, g	1.8	-	1.8	3.3
Cholesterol, mg	-	3	-	-
Calcium, mg	10	3	7	38
Iron, mg	0.53	0.2	1.28	0.69
Phosphorous, mg	77	37	58	54
Magnesium, mg	44	13	18	27
Sodium, mg	1	-	1	36
Potassium, mg	79	29	44	475
Niacin, mg	1.33	0.4	1.689	1.487
Riboflavin, mg	0.012	0.016	0.136	0.106
Vitamin A, IU	-	-	-	19218
Vitamin C, mg	-	-	-	19.6
Vitamin B-6, mg	0.149	0.05	0.049	0.286

Starchy Vegetables, Grains and Breads, serving size 100 grams				
	Corn, Yellow, Raw	Millet, Cooked	Potato, Baked	Quinoa
Water, g	75.96	71.41	74.89	71.61
Calories	86	119	93	120
Carbohydrate*, g	19.02	23.67	21.15	21.3
Protein, g	3.22	3.51	2.5	4.4
Fat, g	1.18	1	0.13	1.92
Fiber, g	2.7	1.3	2.2	2.8
Cholesterol, mg	-	-	-	-
Calcium, mg	2	3	15	17
Iron, mg	0.52	0.63	1.08	1.49
Phosphorous, mg	89	100	70	152
Magnesium, mg	37	44	28	64
Sodium, mg	15	2	10	7
Potassium, mg	270	62	535	172
Niacin, mg	1.7	1.33	1.41	0.412
Riboflavin, mg	0.06	0.082	0.048	0.11
Vitamin A, IU	187	3	10	5
Vitamin C, mg	6.8	-	9.6	-
Vitamin B-6, mg	0.055	0.108	0.311	0.123

More Testimonials

Pam Boteler, Alexandria, Virginia

"When the student is ready, the master appears."

This saying came true for me in August of 2007 when I first met Dr. Doug Graham via e-mail. The last 8 months have just confirmed what I thought prior to meeting him; that is, his work should be required reading for every coaching program in every sport, and required for all athletes, even weekend warriors.

My journey to physical, mental, emotional, and spiritual health hit the speed dial back in August, and I knew I found someone that could help me take my training to a new dimension. Dr. Graham supplied most of the essential ingredients. I merely had to put in the work. At the time we started communicating, I had been vegan for about a year, and prior to that, "mostly" vegetarian for about 4 years, only occasionally eating fish or chicken, as prescribed in "mainstream" circles as mandatory for athletic performance.

Having just come out of yet another major health challenge during the summer of 2007, I was a prime candidate for change. I was "ripe" for a mentor to help me take my health and performance to another level. This was even more poignant for me, being an "older" athlete in a sport where I compete against athletes half my age.

I was pleasantly shocked when Dr. Graham offered to help me in 2007, as I had read about and loosely followed his philosophy and protocol for several years. He quickly learned that I was not only passionate about changing my sport, but also creating new possibilities for my own life and maybe inspiring others in the process. I knew I needed help and recognized that Dr. Graham might just be my missing link.

For the first 2 months, we mostly talked about my sport, performance, and future goals. Then finally, he asked, "Are you ready to get started on 811rv?" I was more than ready and excited. I was at the end of my patience with doctors and "health practitioners" who tried to push medications, supplements, and special diets, including "cleanses," on me to "cure" my ills. And I was tired of blowing A LOT of money on so-called superfood supplements and products. When he told me I was going to spend 7 days on Banana Island, I naively asked, "Where is Banana Island?" I think he gently said, "Right in your own home." I laughed to myself and said, "Okaaaaaay."

I am proud to say I made it through 7 days of Banana Island with only one minor interruption on Day 4, when my second batch of bananas were not ripe enough (as Dr. Graham predicted). I ate grapes to get by, with his permission, and felt like I was cheating! But I did it, consuming 25–30 bananas a day, mostly in smoothie form. I figured I could drink that many—but not eat them.

I actually had one of my highest mileage weeks of the fall in the canoe and had a solid training week overall, and I lost 7 pounds of "waste." For the first time in my life, I lost weight while consuming up to 3,000 calories a day and still maintaining high activity levels. Maybe it was the mental and emotional excitement of working with someone I had only known indirectly through books and speaking. But the physical transformation was remarkable: a physical, mental, and emotional "cleanse" without starvation.

I became hyperaware of the loss of the salt, sugar, and processed tastes I was used to—even those of oils, garlic, and spices. I learned I really didn't need all that to feel satisfied. I learned a big lesson in getting in touch with my body by clearing out the crap and focusing on true physical hunger, even identifying where I should be feeling it (in my throat), and trying to separate emotional, mental, and yes, social hunger from what my body needed.

I will say that week was very difficult and I did complain and get discouraged. But I wanted to do it and was ready because I understood what he was trying to do. Dr. Graham guided me every step of the way, explaining what I was feeling. It was transforming.

Ever since this time and in trying to follow 811rv principles in general, I have to say that this *can be* the simplest formula for success in health and performance, if you are *really* honest with yourself about what your body needs to thrive.

I discovered over time that all this fruit was essentially "nature's candy" and started to appreciate a bigger variety of fruits in my diet. I am not a culinary chef—so simple meals of fruits, even fruit blended with greens into smoothies, have gone a long way to simplify my life and reduce my dependence upon eating out for meals or eating easy to find and cheap-to-buy processed "healthy" foods. Meeting my caloric needs through fruits sounded difficult at first, but has actually become easier with time, even pleasurable. It's just made the most sense. When it has become difficult, it is because *I* have made it difficult. I get in my own way of success!

Even prior to working with Dr. Graham, I felt the incredible power of relying on fruits as my fuel during competitions and as a general rule for pre- and postevent nutrition. I felt, and continue to feel, I can dig deeper and stay "there" longer than ever before, as if there is a new reservoir of energy I can tap into. And, when I am "on" and in a groove, I've recovered from things more quickly and with less soreness. It has been uncanny—but for Dr. Graham—expected business as usual.

Change hasn't happened quickly for me, but slowly I've started to become addicted to THIS phenomenon—the new physical and mental reservoir. When I have briefly gone back to old habits, the reminders are even more painful (physically) than I was used to before. For anyone who has struggled with IBS, as I have, I'm sure you can relate. My taste buds have changed so dramatically as well that most of the foods I used to eat are now just unappealing, if not repulsive.

"Change does not happen until it is more painful not to change"; so, prepare for a metamorphosis.

This is not a "diet," short-term fix, or another fanatical whim— as many around me have "suggested," either directly or indirectly. And it has been difficult socially, but for the most part, people are intrigued and supportive. I have learned to quietly just live this message, rather than trying to explain it, and try not to worry about what people think. If people are interested, then I share what I am experiencing. That has seemed to work, trying to support people where they are and offering encouragement for their path. That seems to work to get food out of the conversation equation and getting the relationship, whatever it may be, in its rightful place back into the equation.

Getting guidance and support from Dr. Graham has gone far beyond food. I know that what I eat creates a stable foundation for my mental, emotional, and spiritual clarity, openness, and general feeling of being grounded and at peace with myself, my relation-ships, and the world. But physically, I have learned the need for adequate—or rather, more—sleep (e.g., I have increased my average nightly sleep by about an hour and could still do more). I learned that in the past, I had not overtrained; I simply underrested—physically, mentally, or emotionally—or all of the above, as was the case in 2007.

I have also, more than ever, realized the importance of sur-rounding myself with more positive and supportive people and thoughts and creating a support structure for myself as I continue on this path and lifestyle. Even my trainer has been 100 percent on board and intrigued since I started. He has been so convinced of the 811rv philosophy that he has applied some of it to his own training protocol and has been preaching these principles to other clients, including his professional athlete clients.

Dr. Graham's philosophy is about so much more than food. And as any athlete knows, so is excelling at one's craft. Your performance and your health are only as strong as your weakest link. It's a package deal—and Dr. Graham and his work are the *real* deal.

Now if all of this could just make my boat go straight....

Dr. Stefania Licari, M.D., London, England

I met Doug a year ago and since then, my approach to nutrition and natural healing has radically changed. Doug showed to me several aspects of the potential of the body to heal itself efficiently and drug free. His approach to a healthy lifestyle is based on years of solid experience and practice, which is the base of a happy, lifelong and injury-free athletic career.

I successfully completed the toughest 150-mile Ultra Marathon in the Amazon jungle in October 2007, and Doug's precious advice about fitness and nutrition played a more-than-crucial role in my success. My overall athletic performance has dramatically improved as well since I have been counting on his constant and reliable support.

Not only is his knowledge a highly recommended asset for any athlete, whether at an amateur or world-class level, but also his ability to offer emotional and mental support for the time pre-, during- and post-races are vital key points.

I am confident that I can count on Dr. Graham's expertise in advising me for all of my fitness and diet endeavors. He is a limitlessly valuable member of my support team for the training preparation of my expeditions.

From running jungle challenges in the Amazon to my incredible self-organized adventure to cover a running distance of more than 1,000 km in North Africa.

Grant Campbell, Sydney, Australia

I'm one of those crazy folk who race alone through remote mountain trails for up to 24 hours on foot, covering distances of 100 km or more. And I do it fueled by low-fat, 100 percent raw-vegan food. No cooking, no heavy processing, no additives. I eat my food 100 percent raw as provided by nature ... no animal cruelty required.

Thanks to Dr. Graham's passion and expertise in sports nutrition, I have the knowledge I require to continue enjoying my trail racing without burning myself out. Having studied Dr. Graham's books, audio, and DVDs, I understand my body's requirements and give myself adequate sleep, rest, sunshine, and fresh air, am always hydrated and ready to race, and no longer suffer cramps or "hit the wall." I finish races feeling fresher than ever before and recover so much faster. I no longer suffer the regular colds and flu that are always "going around." I have increased alertness, mental clarity, endurance, flexibility, and tolerance for the sun (no sunscreen for me). I know what foods and drinks work for my races and how much to consume.

Everything Dr. Graham advocates makes so much sense and works like a dream. I can't recommend his materials strongly enough. Life has so much more to offer when we listen to our bodies and follow the laws of nature. My goal is to run a 100-mile race when I turn 100!

Stefanie Strauss, Costa Mesa, California

Since adopting Dr. Graham's approach as a lifestyle, my fitness and athletic performance have continued to soar.

My endurance has taken on a life of its own, my recoveries are quicker and injury free, my strength is improving. Steadily, my flexibility, agility, and finesse are all moving in the right direction ... forward. I couldn't be more thrilled!

I come from an athletic background which is plagued with numerous injuries. I have "maintained" my fitness for many years, but now with Dr. Graham's advice, I am back in the "game."

Dr. Graham has been so valuable to me in my quest of health and fitness. The best part is that his methods are based on principles of simplicity. When you ask Dr. Graham a question like *"what is the best exercise for shoulders?"* he will smile and tell you ... *"the one that you do."*

He has proven to me there are no secrets to fitness ... he has provided me the tools and laid the foundation for me to train, play, run, jump, and compete. I am having a blast ... and supposedly I am getting older.

ABOUT THE AUTHOR

Dr. Douglas Graham, a raw fooder since the late-'70s, is an advisor to world-class athletes and trainers from around the globe. He has trained professional and Olympic athletes from almost every sport, including tennis legend Martina Navratilova, NBA pro basketball player Ronnie Grandison, Olympic sprinter Doug Dickinson, and professional golfer Aree Song. In addition, Dr. Graham has worked with the United States Olympic Diving team, the Norwegian National Bicycling team and many other Olympian and professional athletes. Models, actors, physicians, performers, and motivated people from all walks of life have sought his inspiration and guidance as a health coach. Mark Victor Hansen, co-author of the *Chicken Soup for the Soul* series, is one of his long-term clients. Anthony Robbins and Harvey Diamond are both supporters of his work.

Dr. Graham's ability to reach a mainstream audience with a healthy raw food message has brought thousands of people into the health movement. His importance to the movement can best be expressed by noting that he has given the keynote address at every major raw food event, worldwide, since 1998. Dr. Graham's boundless energy and joy for living is definitely contagious. A professional speaker since 1979, Dr. Graham seeks to make a point while making a friend, congratulating people for what they have achieved, and motivating them to strive for more. He has given more than 5,000 presentations during his illustrious career.

Dr. Graham is the author of *The NEW High Energy Diet Recipe Guide, The Perpetual Health Calendar, Nutrition and Athletic Performance,*

Hygienic Fasting, The 80/10/10 Diet, and *Grain Damage.* He has shared his strategies for achieving optimum health with audiences at events sponsored by the International College of Integrative Medicine; the American, British, and Canadian Natural Hygiene Societies; the North American, European, and World Vegetarian Societies; the American and British Vegan Societies; EarthSave International; Fitness Professionals U.K.; the American Fruitarian Society; The Essenes; Vitalities Inc.; Living Light Culinary Arts Institute; and many others. He is a regular speaker at many national and international health, animal rights, environmental, and sports performance seminars. Dr. Graham has given presentations for many of the world's chiropractic colleges and has spoken at a variety of college campuses around the world.

Dr. Graham was in private practice as a chiropractor for 20 years and was the owner and director of Club Hygiene, a fasting retreat in the Florida Keys, for 10 of those years. He also served on the board of governors of the International Association of Professional Natural Hygienists and the board of directors of the American Natural Hygiene Society. He was a founder of Healthful Living International, the world's only international Natural Hygiene organization, where he served three consecutive terms. He is on the board of advisors for the Vegetarian Union of North America, Voice for a Viable Future, Living Light Films, The Society of Ethical and Religious Vegetarians, Ekaya Institute, and EarthSave International. He also serves as nutrition advisor for the magazine, *Exercise, For Men Only.* He is raw foods and fitness advisor for VegSource.com, the largest vegetarian Web site on the Internet, and he taught the Health Educators program at Hippocrates Institute. In addition, he served as the "source authority" for the Harmonious Living Web site and has authored regular columns for *Fresh Network* magazine, *Just Eat an Apple* magazine, *Ficus* magazine, and *Living Nutrition/Vibrance* magazine. In addition to working on his next book, Dr. Graham currently also writes columns for *Primal Parenting* magazine and *Flying Disc* magazine.

RECOMMENDED READING LIST

Allen, Hannah, *The Happy Truth about Protein,* by Life Science, 1972

Berry, Rynn, *Food for the Gods: Vegetarianism & the World's Religions,* Pythagorean Publishers, 1998

Bowsher, David, *Introduction to the Anatomy and Physiology of the Nervous System,* Year Book Medical Pub; 4th edition, 1979

Calabro, Rose Lee, *Living in the Raw,* Book Publishing Company, 2003

Coleman, John, *Opioids in Common Food Products: Addictive Peptides in Meat, Dairy and Grains,* 1995

Devries, Herbert A.; Loree L. Weir; Terry J. Housh, *Physiology of Exercise for Physical Education, Athletics, Exercise Science,* Brown and Benchmark Pub, 1995

Dye, Michael, and George Malkmus, *God's Way to Ultimate Health,* Hallelujah Acres Publishing, 2004

Fry, Terry C., *Better Sleep for a Better Life,* Life Science Society, 1970

Fry, Terry, C., and Essie Honiball, *I Live On Fruit,* Life Science Institute, 1991

Fry, Terry C., and David Klein, *Your Natural Diet: Alive Raw Foods,* Living Nutrition Publications, 2004

Goldburg, Burton; John W. Anderson; Larry Trivieri, *Alternative Medicine,* Ten Speed Press, 2002

Graham, Douglas N., *Grain Damage,* FoodnSport Press, 2007

Graham, Douglas N., *The High Energy Diet Nutrition Food Combining Chart,* FoodnSport Press, 2001

Graham, Douglas N., *The New High Energy Diet Recipe Guide,* FoodnSport Press, 2007

Gray, Henry, *Anatomy, Descriptive and Surgical,* Bounty Books, 1977

Guthrie, Helen Andrews, *Introductory Nutrition, Mosby Year Book,* 1988

Immerman, Alan M., *Health Unlimited,* Naturegraph Publishers, 1990

Johnson, Perry, and Donald Stolberg, *Conditioning,* Prentice Hall, 1971

Kenton, Leslie, and Susannah, Kenton, *Raw Energy,* Warner Books, 1986

Leakey, Richard, *The Origin of Humankind,* Basic Books, 1996

Leonardo, Blanche, *Cancer and Other Diseases Caused by Meat Consumption,* Tree of Life Publications, 1985

Lyman, Howard F., and Glen Merzer, *Mad Cowboy,* Scribner, 2001

Mackenna, Ann B., and Robin Callander, *Illustrated Physiology,* Churchhill Livingstone; 6th edition, 1997

McMinn, R. M. H., *The Human Gut,* Oxford University Press, 1974

Nelson, Dennis, *Food Combining Simplified,* Publisher Dennis Nelson, 1988

O. L. M., *Fruit Can Heal You,* Nutritional and Natural Health Publications, 1981

Paavo, Airola, *How to Get Well,* Health Plus Publishers, 1974

Pickering, Wayne, *The Perfect Diet,* 1980

Shelton, Herbert M., *Food Combining Made Easy,* Willow Publishing, 1982

Shelton, Herbert M., *Orthopathy,* Dr. Shelton's Health School, 1939

Shelton, Herbert M., *The Myth of Medicine,* Cool Hand Communications Inc., 1995

Shelton, Herbert M., *The Science and Fine Art of Food and Nutrition,* National Health Association; 6th edition, 1984

Stanley, Tyler, *Diet by Design,* Teach Services, Inc., 1998

Wells, Katharine F., *Kinesiology,* William C Brown Pub; 7th edition, 1989

Williams, Clyde, and John T. Devlin, (Eds.), *Foods, Nutrition and Sports Performance,* Taylor & Francis, 1992

Williams, Thomas R., *The Laws of Vital Relation,* 1985

Wilson, Edward O., *Biophilia,* Harvard University Press, 1986